DIPHENHYDRAMINE

A MEDICAL DICTIONARY, BIBLIOGRAPHY,
AND ANNOTATED RESEARCH GUIDE TO
INTERNET REFERENCES

JAMES N. PARKER, M.D.
AND PHILIP M. PARKER, PH.D., EDITORS

ICON Health Publications
ICON Group International, Inc.
4370 La Jolla Village Drive, 4th Floor
San Diego, CA 92122 USA

Last digit indicates print number: 10 9 8 7 6 4 5 3 2 1

Publisher, Health Care: Philip Parker, Ph.D.
Editor(s): James Parker, M.D., Philip Parker, Ph.D.

Publisher's note: The ideas, procedures, and suggestions contained in this book are not intended for the diagnosis or treatment of a health problem. As new medical or scientific information becomes available from academic and clinical research, recommended treatments and drug therapies may undergo changes. The authors, editors, and publisher have attempted to make the information in this book up to date and accurate in accord with accepted standards at the time of publication. The authors, editors, and publisher are not responsible for errors or omissions or for consequences from application of the book, and make no warranty, expressed or implied, in regard to the contents of this book. Any practice described in this book should be applied by the reader in accordance with professional standards of care used in regard to the unique circumstances that may apply in each situation. The reader is advised to always check product information (package inserts) for changes and new information regarding dosage and contraindications before prescribing any drug or pharmacological product. Caution is especially urged when using new or infrequently ordered drugs, herbal remedies, vitamins and supplements, alternative therapies, complementary therapies and medicines, and integrative medical treatments.

Cataloging-in-Publication Data

Parker, James N., 1961-
Parker, Philip M., 1960-

     Diphenhydramine: A Medical Dictionary, Bibliography, and Annotated Research Guide to Internet References /
James N. Parker and Philip M. Parker, editors
          p.   cm.
     Includes bibliographical references, glossary, and index.
     ISBN: 0-497-00369-4
     1. Diphenhydramine-Popular works. I. Title.

Disclaimer

This publication is not intended to be used for the diagnosis or treatment of a health problem. It is sold with the understanding that the publisher, editors, and authors are not engaging in the rendering of medical, psychological, financial, legal, or other professional services.

References to any entity, product, service, or source of information that may be contained in this publication should not be considered an endorsement, either direct or implied, by the publisher, editors, or authors. ICON Group International, Inc., the editors, and the authors are not responsible for the content of any Web pages or publications referenced in this publication.

Copyright Notice

Acknowledgements

The collective knowledge generated from academic and applied research summarized in various references has been critical in the creation of this book which is best viewed as a comprehensive compilation and collection of information prepared by various official agencies which produce publications on diphenhydramine. Books in this series draw from various agencies and institutions associated with the United States Department of Health and Human Services, and in particular, the Office of the Secretary of Health and Human Services (OS), the Administration for Children and Families (ACF), the Administration on Aging (AOA), the Agency for Healthcare Research and Quality (AHRQ), the Agency for Toxic Substances and Disease Registry (ATSDR), the Centers for Disease Control and Prevention (CDC), the Food and Drug Administration (FDA), the Healthcare Financing Administration (HCFA), the Health Resources and Services Administration (HRSA), the Indian Health Service (IHS), the institutions of the National Institutes of Health (NIH), the Program Support Center (PSC), and the Substance Abuse and Mental Health Services Administration (SAMHSA). In addition to these sources, information gathered from the National Library of Medicine, the United States Patent Office, the European Union, and their related organizations has been invaluable in the creation of this book. Some of the work represented was financially supported by the Research and Development Committee at INSEAD. This support is gratefully acknowledged. Finally, special thanks are owed to Tiffany Freeman for her excellent editorial support.

About the Editors

James N. Parker, M.D.

Dr. James N. Parker received his Bachelor of Science degree in Psychobiology from the University of California, Riverside and his M.D. from the University of California, San Diego. In addition to authoring numerous research publications, he has lectured at various academic institutions. Dr. Parker is the medical editor for health books by ICON Health Publications.

Philip M. Parker, Ph.D.

Philip M. Parker is the Eli Lilly Chair Professor of Innovation, Business and Society at INSEAD (Fontainebleau, France and Singapore). Dr. Parker has also been Professor at the University of California, San Diego and has taught courses at Harvard University, the Hong Kong University of Science and Technology, the Massachusetts Institute of Technology, Stanford University, and UCLA. Dr. Parker is the associate editor for ICON Health Publications.

About ICON Health Publications

To discover more about ICON Health Publications, simply check with your preferred online booksellers, including Barnes&Noble.com and Amazon.com which currently carry all of our titles. Or, feel free to contact us directly for bulk purchases or institutional discounts:

ICON Group International, Inc.
4370 La Jolla Village Drive, Fourth Floor
San Diego, CA 92122 USA
Fax: 858-546-4341
Web site: **www.icongrouponline.com/health**

Table of Contents

FORWARD

In March 2001, the National Institutes of Health issued the following warning: "The number of Web sites offering health-related resources grows every day. Many sites provide valuable information, while others may have information that is unreliable or misleading."[1] Furthermore, because of the rapid increase in Internet-based information, many hours can be wasted searching, selecting, and printing. Since only the smallest fraction of information dealing with diphenhydramine is indexed in search engines, such as **www.google.com** or others, a non-systematic approach to Internet research can be not only time consuming, but also incomplete. This book was created for medical professionals, students, and members of the general public who want to know as much as possible about diphenhydramine, using the most advanced research tools available and spending the least amount of time doing so.

In addition to offering a structured and comprehensive bibliography, the pages that follow will tell you where and how to find reliable information covering virtually all topics related to diphenhydramine, from the essentials to the most advanced areas of research. Public, academic, government, and peer-reviewed research studies are emphasized. Various abstracts are reproduced to give you some of the latest official information available to date on diphenhydramine. Abundant guidance is given on how to obtain free-of-charge primary research results via the Internet. **While this book focuses on the field of medicine, when some sources provide access to non-medical information relating to diphenhydramine, these are noted in the text.**

E-book and electronic versions of this book are fully interactive with each of the Internet sites mentioned (clicking on a hyperlink automatically opens your browser to the site indicated). If you are using the hard copy version of this book, you can access a cited Web site by typing the provided Web address directly into your Internet browser. You may find it useful to refer to synonyms or related terms when accessing these Internet databases. **NOTE:** At the time of publication, the Web addresses were functional. However, some links may fail due to URL address changes, which is a common occurrence on the Internet.

For readers unfamiliar with the Internet, detailed instructions are offered on how to access electronic resources. For readers unfamiliar with medical terminology, a comprehensive glossary is provided. For readers without access to Internet resources, a directory of medical libraries, that have or can locate references cited here, is given. We hope these resources will prove useful to the widest possible audience seeking information on diphenhydramine.

The Editors

---

[1] From the NIH, National Cancer Institute (NCI): **http://www.cancer.gov/cancerinfo/ten-things-to-know**.

CHAPTER 1. STUDIES ON DIPHENHYDRAMINE

Overview

In this chapter, we will show you how to locate peer-reviewed references and studies on diphenhydramine.

The Combined Health Information Database

The Combined Health Information Database summarizes studies across numerous federal agencies. To limit your investigation to research studies and diphenhydramine, you will need to use the advanced search options. First, go to **http://chid.nih.gov/index.html**. From there, select the "Detailed Search" option (or go directly to that page with the following hyperlink: **http://chid.nih.gov/detail/detail.html**). The trick in extracting studies is found in the drop boxes at the bottom of the search page where "You may refine your search by." Select the dates and language you prefer, and the format option "Journal Article." At the top of the search form, select the number of records you would like to see (we recommend 100) and check the box to display "whole records." We recommend that you type "diphenhydramine" (or synonyms) into the "For these words:" box. Consider using the option "anywhere in record" to make your search as broad as possible. If you want to limit the search to only a particular field, such as the title of the journal, then select this option in the "Search in these fields" drop box. The following is what you can expect from this type of search:

- **Pharmacologic Treatment of Noncognitive Behavioral Disturbances in Elderly Demented Patients**

  Source: American Journal of Psychiatry. 147(12): 1640-1645. December 1990.

  Summary: Fifty-nine elderly residents of long-term care facilities who had DSM-II diagnoses of dementia were studied in an 8-week randomized, double-blind comparison trial of haloperidol, oxazepam, and **diphenhydramine** to test the efficacy of these agents in the treatment of clinically significant behavioral disturbances in patients with dementia. All three agents demonstrated modest but significant efficacy as measured by clinical ratings of agitated behavior and activities of daily living. The absolute magnitude of improvement was greater for haloperidol and **diphenhydramine** than for oxazepam, but differences among groups did not approach statistical significance. Frequencies of acute adverse events during the trial were similar across the drug treatment groups. Although these drugs may differ in terms of long-term safety and efficacy, they appear to be equivalent for short-term management of agitated behavior in severely demented patients. 32 references. (AA).

- **Medical Treatment of Meniere's Disease**

Source: Otolaryngologic Clinics of North America. 30(6): 1027-1037. December 1997.

Summary: Meniere's disease is an idiopathic disease involving the inner ear that is characterized by vertigo, hearing loss, and tinnitus. The hearing loss is fluctuating, usually low-frequency, sensorineural in type, and associated with tinnitus (ringing or buzzing in the ears). This article reviews the drug therapy used in treating Meniere's disease. The authors first discuss the treatment of acute labyrinthine crisis, including medications that provide relief to patients of the nausea, vomiting, and vertigo that accompanies the acute attack. Although these medications provide symptomatic relief, they are not thought to reverse the original pathologic process of Meniere's disease but only control the symptoms. The second half of the article discusses medications used to help prevent attacks of Meniere's disease. Nonsurgical treatment of Meniere's disease is considered effective in approximately 80 percent of Meniere's disease patients and forms the primary mode of therapy in managing these patients. Drugs to treat acute episodes include diazepam (Valium), anticholinergic drugs (glycopyrrolate), antidopaminergic drugs (droperidol and prochlorperazine), and antihistamines (dimenhydrinate, **diphenhydramine,** meclizine, promethazine). Maintenance therapy can include diet modifications, diuretics (including thiazide diuretics), and carbonic anhydrase inhibitors. Ablative therapy can include aminoglycosides (which are ototoxic). Other medications used can include vasodilators, calcium channel blockers, ACE inhibitors, lipoflavins, and vitamins. The authors conclude that the therapeutic efficacy of drugs used to manage vertigo associated with this disorder is difficult to evaluate because spontaneous remission may occur. 2 tables. 19 references.

- **Single-Case-Study Method for Treating Resistiveness in Patients With Alzheimer's Disease**

Source: Hospital and Community Psychiatry. 43(7): 720-724. July 1992.

Summary: This journal article describes a single case study approach to identify the best medication for treating resistiveness to care in patients with moderate dementia. Using a double blind research design, the researchers devised a four point resistiveness rating scale, ranging from no resistiveness to severe resistiveness. Specific behaviors associated with each of the four stages of resistiveness are described. Three medications, randomly labeled, were administered in series of trials in 1 week blocks. The medication trials, baselines, patient resistiveness ratings by nurses, and visual and statistical analysis of the results were examined to determine the drug that provided the most stable response at the lowest dose. In the six patients who completed the trial, thiothixene was found to be more effective than oxazepam and **diphenhydramine.** Discussions about the implications of patient behavior on drug administration and dosage and the use of this type of study design for future research are included. 13 references.

- **When Your Stomach Complains**

Source: Healthline. 18(11): 8-9. November 1999.

Contact: Available from Healthline Publishing, Inc. 830 Menlo Avenue, Suite 100, Menlo Park, CA 94025. (650) 325-6457. Website: www.healthline.com.

Summary: This newsletter article offers an indepth look at nausea, vomiting and heartburn. The author focuses on the use of drugs to treat motion sickness and heartburn. The first section addresses motion sickness, noting that the primary culprit in this condition is excess stimulation to the inner ear's maze of fluid filled canals, responsible for maintaining the body's balance. Poor ventilation, anxiety or other emotional upset, and visual stimuli may contribute to motion sickness. The author recommends preventive treatment, with the use of an over the counter (OTC) drug taken 30 to 60 minutes before traveling. The drugs considered to be safe and effective for use in OTC drugs for motion sickness are: cyclizine (Marezine and others), dimenhydrinate (Dramamine and others), **diphenhydramine** (Benadryl and others), and meclizine (Bonine and others). The author briefly reviews factors to be considered when using these medications. The second section on heartburn discusses four OTC drugs, Pepcid AC Acid Controller (famotidine), Tagamet HB (cimetidine), Axid AR (nizatidine), and Zantac 75 (ranitidine hydrochloride), that work systematically to reduce the amount of stomach acid produced. The author also discusses products approved to relieve heartburn, indigestion or upset stomach from too much food or drink, i.e., antacids, which neutralize gastric acidity. The four general categories are discussed, with common brands and potential side effects: sodium salts (Alka Seltzer, Bromo Seltzer), calcium salts (Alka 2, Rolaids, Tums), aluminum salts (ALTernaGEL, Amphojel, Rolaids), and magnesium salts (Camalox, Gelusil, Maalox, Mylanta). The article concludes with a brief discussion of the role of overindulgence, viral infection, and some general advice. One sidebar lists ways to avoid heartburn.

Federally Funded Research on Diphenhydramine

The U.S. Government supports a variety of research studies relating to diphenhydramine. These studies are tracked by the Office of Extramural Research at the National Institutes of Health.[2] CRISP (Computerized Retrieval of Information on Scientific Projects) is a searchable database of federally funded biomedical research projects conducted at universities, hospitals, and other institutions.

Search the CRISP Web site at **http://crisp.cit.nih.gov/crisp/crisp_query.generate_screen**. You will have the option to perform targeted searches by various criteria, including geography, date, and topics related to diphenhydramine.

For most of the studies, the agencies reporting into CRISP provide summaries or abstracts. As opposed to clinical trial research using patients, many federally funded studies use animals or simulated models to explore diphenhydramine. The following is typical of the type of information found when searching the CRISP database for diphenhydramine:

- **Project Title: NEUROCOGNITIVE ASSESSMENT SYSTEM FOR THE ELDERLY**

  Principal Investigator & Institution: Gevins, Alan S.; President; Sam Technology, Inc. 425 Bush St, 5Th Fl San Francisco, Ca 94108

  Timing: Fiscal Year 2002; Project Start 01-APR-1999; Project End 31-AUG-2005

---

[2] Healthcare projects are funded by the National Institutes of Health (NIH), Substance Abuse and Mental Health Services (SAMHSA), Health Resources and Services Administration (HRSA), Food and Drug Administration (FDA), Centers for Disease Control and Prevention (CDCP), Agency for Healthcare Research and Quality (AHRQ), and Office of Assistant Secretary of Health (OASH).

Summary: (provided by applicant): Many medical treatments produce subtle changes in working and intermediate term memory and executive functioning in the elderly. Some medical treatments may have negative cognitive side effects, whereas other treatments improve cognitive function. Prior work demonstrates that combinations of EEG, event related potential and cognitive task performance data are sensitive and specific indicators of level of alertness and ability to sustain attention and hold information in working and intermediate term memory. We propose to develop a specialized automated device utilizing multivariate combinations of these measures to detect treatment related changes in neurocognitive function in the elderly. In Phase I feasibility was evaluated by analyzing task performance and EEG data from elderly subjects after they ingested a common OTC drug, the antihistamine **diphenhydramine.** We computed multivariate indices from these data, and determined that they could discriminate post-drug conditions from placebo. Additionally, we identified improvements required for use of our automated task presentation and signal processing algorithms with elderly subjects, and designed modifications to a system for administering, analyzing and tracking tests and results. In Phase II, the system will be fully implemented and independently tested in collaboration with scientists and clinicians at four university medical centers. PROPOSED COMMERCIAL APPLICATION: The proposed system will enable researchers to better evaluate how medical treatments affect neurocognitive function in the elderly. The market for such a device is sufficient to sustain the product. The system may also prove clinically useful as a means for titrating drug dosages and for tracking neurocognitive changes in the treatment of individual patients. Thus, a second-generation device may serve as a more general clinical tool for monitoring changes in cognitive status in the elderly. There is a large and rapidly growing market for such a clinical device.

Website: http://crisp.cit.nih.gov/crisp/Crisp_Query.Generate_Screen

- **Project Title: POLYSOMNOGRAPHIC ASSESSMENT OF ALTERNATIVE TREATMENT**

Principal Investigator & Institution: Bliwise, Donald L.; Professor; Neurology; Emory University 1784 North Decatur Road Atlanta, Ga 30322

Timing: Fiscal Year 2002; Project Start 01-SEP-2000; Project End 30-JUN-2005

Summary: Patients with Parkinson's Disease have exceptionally poor sleep. Even relative to other neurodegenerative diseases such as Alzheimer's Disease, the sleep of the PD patient is fragmented and disturbed. Most notably, sleep in PD is characterized by excessive activity in surface electomyographic (EMG) recordings from many different muscle groups. Despite the sleep disturbance, approximately 50 percent of PD patients note that, on nights when they are able to achieve sleep, they experience a transient (1 to 3 hour) reduction in waking motor symptoms upon arising in the morning. This effect has been termed Sleep Benefit. To date there are no double-blind placebo-controlled studies treating sleep disturbance using PD using any (conventional or alternative) medical treatments. In this randomized, double- blind, parallel-groups, placebo-controlled polysomnographic clinical trial we will compare two alternative medical treatments (valerian, melatonin) and two conventional medical treatments (diphenhydramine, zolpidem) for the disturbed sleep of PD patients. Compelling basic science and clinical rationales exist for use of each of these substances (including valerian and melatonin) for treatment of sleep disturbance in PD. The proposed study will be conducted for six consecutive nights (3 Baseline, 3 Drug) using state-of the-art digitized ambulatory polysomnography in each patient's home. Outcomes will include both measures of nocturnal sleep and waking motor function. Polysomnographic measurements will include customary variables such as total sleep time, sleep efficiency and sleep latency, as well as EMG measures of periodic and isolated muscle activity during sleep. Assessments of motor function will be made the morning immediately, following the third Baseline night and third Drug night in order to test for improvement related to improved sleep. Data will be analyzed with Analysis of Covariance examining Condition (Baseline, Drug), (valerian, melatonin, **diphenhydramine,** zolpidem, placebo), and characteristic Sleep Benefit (positive, negative) main effects, as well as their interactions, after adjusting for Baseline values. The results would represent the first data applying rigorous clinical trial methodology to the study of disturbance sleep in PD patients and would critically examine the efficacy of two substances currently seeing widespread use as over-the counter hypnotics for which little polysomnographic data currently exist.

Website: http://crisp.cit.nih.gov/crisp/Crisp_Query.Generate_Screen

E-Journals: PubMed Central[3]

PubMed Central (PMC) is a digital archive of life sciences journal literature developed and managed by the National Center for Biotechnology Information (NCBI) at the U.S. National Library of Medicine (NLM).[4] Access to this growing archive of e-journals is free and unrestricted.[5] To search, go to **http://www.ncbi.nlm.nih.gov/entrez/query.fcgi?db=Pmc**, and type "diphenhydramine" (or synonyms) into the search box. This search gives you access to full-text articles. The following is a sample of items found for diphenhydramine in the PubMed Central database:

- **Effects of antihistamines on the lung vascular response to histamine in unanesthetized sheep. Diphenhydramine prevention of pulmonary edema and increased permeability.** by Brigham KL, Bowers RE, Owen PJ.; 1976 Aug;
  http://www.pubmedcentral.gov/picrender.fcgi?tool=pmcentrez&action=stream&blobtype=pdf&artid=333194

The National Library of Medicine: PubMed

One of the quickest and most comprehensive ways to find academic studies in both English and other languages is to use PubMed, maintained by the National Library of Medicine.[6] The advantage of PubMed over previously mentioned sources is that it covers a greater number of domestic and foreign references. It is also free to use. If the publisher has a Web site that offers full text of its journals, PubMed will provide links to that site, as well as to

---

[3] Adapted from the National Library of Medicine: **http://www.pubmedcentral.nih.gov/about/intro.html**.

[4] With PubMed Central, NCBI is taking the lead in preservation and maintenance of open access to electronic literature, just as NLM has done for decades with printed biomedical literature. PubMed Central aims to become a world-class library of the digital age.

[5] The value of PubMed Central, in addition to its role as an archive, lies in the availability of data from diverse sources stored in a common format in a single repository. Many journals already have online publishing operations, and there is a growing tendency to publish material online only, to the exclusion of print.

[6] PubMed was developed by the National Center for Biotechnology Information (NCBI) at the National Library of Medicine (NLM) at the National Institutes of Health (NIH). The PubMed database was developed in conjunction with publishers of biomedical literature as a search tool for accessing literature citations and linking to full-text journal articles at Web sites of participating publishers. Publishers that participate in PubMed supply NLM with their citations electronically prior to or at the time of publication.

sites offering other related data. User registration, a subscription fee, or some other type of fee may be required to access the full text of articles in some journals.

To generate your own bibliography of studies dealing with diphenhydramine, simply go to the PubMed Web site at **http://www.ncbi.nlm.nih.gov/pubmed**. Type "diphenhydramine" (or synonyms) into the search box, and click "Go." The following is the type of output you can expect from PubMed for diphenhydramine (hyperlinks lead to article summaries):

- **1% lidocaine versus 0.5% diphenhydramine for local anesthesia in minor laceration repair.**
  Author(s): Ernst AA, Marvez-Valls E, Mall G, Patterson J, Xie X, Weiss SJ.
  Source: Annals of Emergency Medicine. 1994 June; 23(6): 1328-32.
  http://www.ncbi.nlm.nih.gov/entrez/query.fcgi?cmd=Retrieve&db=pubmed&dopt=Abstract&list_uids=8198309

- **A case of massive diphenhydramine abuse and withdrawal from use of the drug.**
  Author(s): Feldman MD, Behar M.
  Source: Jama : the Journal of the American Medical Association. 1986 June 13; 255(22): 3119-20.
  http://www.ncbi.nlm.nih.gov/entrez/query.fcgi?cmd=Retrieve&db=pubmed&dopt=Abstract&list_uids=3702020

- **A comparison of assessment techniques measuring the effects of methylphenidate, secobarbital, diazepam and diphenhydramine in abstinent alcoholics.**
  Author(s): Miller TP, Taylor JL, Tinklenberg JR.
  Source: Neuropsychobiology. 1988; 19(2): 90-6.
  http://www.ncbi.nlm.nih.gov/entrez/query.fcgi?cmd=Retrieve&db=pubmed&dopt=Abstract&list_uids=3226529

- **A comparison of methods for assessing the sedative effects of diphenhydramine on skills related to car driving.**
  Author(s): Cohen AF, Posner J, Ashby L, Smith R, Peck AW.
  Source: European Journal of Clinical Pharmacology. 1984; 27(4): 477-82.
  http://www.ncbi.nlm.nih.gov/entrez/query.fcgi?cmd=Retrieve&db=pubmed&dopt=Abstract&list_uids=6519156

- **A comparison of the effect of diphenhydramine and desloratadine on vigilance and cognitive function during treatment of ragweed-induced allergic rhinitis.**
  Author(s): Wilken JA, Kane RL, Ellis AK, Rafeiro E, Briscoe MP, Sullivan CL, Day JH.
  Source: Annals of Allergy, Asthma & Immunology : Official Publication of the American College of Allergy, Asthma, & Immunology. 2003 October; 91(4): 375-85.
  http://www.ncbi.nlm.nih.gov/entrez/query.fcgi?cmd=Retrieve&db=pubmed&dopt=Abstract&list_uids=14582817

- **A double-blind clinical trial on diphenhydramine in pertussis.**
  Author(s): Danzon A, Lacroix J, Infante-Rivard C, Chicoine L.
  Source: Acta Paediatr Scand. 1988 July; 77(4): 614-5. No Abstract Available.
  http://www.ncbi.nlm.nih.gov/entrez/query.fcgi?cmd=Retrieve&db=pubmed&dopt=Abstract&list_uids=3293352

- A double-blind comparison of oxatomide (R 35 443) and diphenhydramine in the treatment of hay fever.
  Author(s): van der Bijl WJ, Cordier R, van Dishoeck EA, De Proost W, Vannieuwenhuyse E.
  Source: The Laryngoscope. 1980 January; 90(1): 145-51.
  http://www.ncbi.nlm.nih.gov/entrez/query.fcgi?cmd=Retrieve&db=pubmed&dopt=Abstract&list_uids=6986007

- A pilot study of metoclopramide, dexamethasone, diphenhydramine and lorazepam in prevention of nausea and vomiting in cisplatin-treated male patients.
  Author(s): Roila F, Basurto C, Bracarda S, Picciafuoco M, Ballatori E, Del Favero A, Tonato M.
  Source: Oncology. 1990; 47(5): 415-7.
  http://www.ncbi.nlm.nih.gov/entrez/query.fcgi?cmd=Retrieve&db=pubmed&dopt=Abstract&list_uids=2216296

- A randomised, double-blind comparison of granisetron with high-dose metoclopramide, dexamethasone and diphenhydramine for cisplatin-induced emesis. An NCI Canada Clinical Trials Group Phase III Trial.
  Author(s): Warr D, Wilan A, Venner P, Pater J, Kaizer L, Laberge F, Latreille J, Stewart D, O'Connell G, Osoba D, et al.
  Source: European Journal of Cancer (Oxford, England : 1990). 1992; 29A(1): 33-6.
  http://www.ncbi.nlm.nih.gov/entrez/query.fcgi?cmd=Retrieve&db=pubmed&dopt=Abstract&list_uids=1332737

- A rapid and sensitive spectrophotometric procedure for the determination of diphenhydramine and related ethers.
  Author(s): Caddy B, Fish F, Tranter J.
  Source: The Analyst. 1975 August; 100(1193): 563-6.
  http://www.ncbi.nlm.nih.gov/entrez/query.fcgi?cmd=Retrieve&db=pubmed&dopt=Abstract&list_uids=1163792

- A study of the plasma levels of pentaerythritol mononitrate following administration of pentaerythritol tetranitrate in combination with meprobamate and diphenhydramine.
  Author(s): Gilbert JD, Aylott RI, Draffan GH, Sogtrop HH.
  Source: Arzneimittel-Forschung. 1982; 32(5): 571-4.
  http://www.ncbi.nlm.nih.gov/entrez/query.fcgi?cmd=Retrieve&db=pubmed&dopt=Abstract&list_uids=7201836

- A trial of Lotussin and linctus diphenhydramine in patients wth an irritant cough.
  Author(s): Matts SG.
  Source: J Int Med Res. 1977; 5(6): 470-2.
  http://www.ncbi.nlm.nih.gov/entrez/query.fcgi?cmd=Retrieve&db=pubmed&dopt=Abstract&list_uids=338397

- **Absence of pharmacokinetic interaction between orally co-administered naproxen sodium and diphenhydramine hydrochloride.**
  Author(s): Toothaker RD, Barker SH, Gillen MV, Helsinger SA, Kindberg CG, Hunt TL, Powell JH.
  Source: Biopharmaceutics & Drug Disposition. 2000 September; 21(6): 229-33.
  http://www.ncbi.nlm.nih.gov/entrez/query.fcgi?cmd=Retrieve&db=pubmed&dopt=Abstract&list_uids=11304721

- **Abuse liability of diphenhydramine in sedative abusers.**
  Author(s): Wolf B, Guarino JJ, Preston KL, Griffiths RR.
  Source: Nida Res Monogr. 1989; 95: 486-7. No Abstract Available.
  http://www.ncbi.nlm.nih.gov/entrez/query.fcgi?cmd=Retrieve&db=pubmed&dopt=Abstract&list_uids=2577046

- **Abuse potential of methaqualone-diphenhydramine combination.**
  Author(s): Coleman JB, Barcone JA.
  Source: Am J Hosp Pharm. 1981 February; 38(2): 160. No Abstract Available.
  http://www.ncbi.nlm.nih.gov/entrez/query.fcgi?cmd=Retrieve&db=pubmed&dopt=Abstract&list_uids=7211878

- **Accidental childhood death from diphenhydramine overdosage.**
  Author(s): Goetz CM, Lopez G, Dean BS, Krenzelok EP.
  Source: The American Journal of Emergency Medicine. 1990 July; 8(4): 321-2.
  http://www.ncbi.nlm.nih.gov/entrez/query.fcgi?cmd=Retrieve&db=pubmed&dopt=Abstract&list_uids=2363755

- **Acetaminophen and diphenhydramine as premedication for platelet transfusions: a prospective randomized double-blind placebo-controlled trial.**
  Author(s): Wang SE, Lara PN Jr, Lee-Ow A, Reed J, Wang LR, Palmer P, Tuscano JM, Richman CM, Beckett L, Wun T.
  Source: American Journal of Hematology. 2002 July; 70(3): 191-4.
  http://www.ncbi.nlm.nih.gov/entrez/query.fcgi?cmd=Retrieve&db=pubmed&dopt=Abstract&list_uids=12111764

- **Acrivastine, terfenadine and diphenhydramine effects on driving performance as a function of dose and time after dosing.**
  Author(s): Ramaekers JG, O'Hanlon JF.
  Source: European Journal of Clinical Pharmacology. 1994; 47(3): 261-6.
  http://www.ncbi.nlm.nih.gov/entrez/query.fcgi?cmd=Retrieve&db=pubmed&dopt=Abstract&list_uids=7867679

- **Activated charcoal adsorption of diphenhydramine.**
  Author(s): Guay DR, Meatherall RC, Macaulay PA, Yeung C.
  Source: Int J Clin Pharmacol Ther Toxicol. 1984 August; 22(8): 395-400.
  http://www.ncbi.nlm.nih.gov/entrez/query.fcgi?cmd=Retrieve&db=pubmed&dopt=Abstract&list_uids=6490221

- **Acute and subacute actions on human performance and interactions with diazepam of temelastine (SK&F93944) and diphenhydramine.**
  Author(s): Mattila MJ, Mattila M, Konno K.
  Source: European Journal of Clinical Pharmacology. 1986; 31(3): 291-8.
  http://www.ncbi.nlm.nih.gov/entrez/query.fcgi?cmd=Retrieve&db=pubmed&dopt=Abstract&list_uids=2878812

- **Acute and subchronic effects of levocetirizine and diphenhydramine on memory functioning, psychomotor performance, and mood.**
  Author(s): Verster JC, Volkerts ER, van Oosterwijck AW, Aarab M, Bijtjes SI, De Weert AM, Eijken EJ, Verbaten MN.
  Source: The Journal of Allergy and Clinical Immunology. 2003 March; 111(3): 623-7.
  http://www.ncbi.nlm.nih.gov/entrez/query.fcgi?cmd=Retrieve&db=pubmed&dopt=Abstract&list_uids=12642847

- **Acute delirium associated with combined diphenhydramine and linezolid use.**
  Author(s): Serio RN.
  Source: The Annals of Pharmacotherapy. 2004 January; 38(1): 62-5.
  http://www.ncbi.nlm.nih.gov/entrez/query.fcgi?cmd=Retrieve&db=pubmed&dopt=Abstract&list_uids=14742796

- **Acute dystonia. An unusal reaction to diphenhydramine.**
  Author(s): Lavenstein BL, Cantor FK.
  Source: Jama : the Journal of the American Medical Association. 1976 July 19; 236(3): 291.
  http://www.ncbi.nlm.nih.gov/entrez/query.fcgi?cmd=Retrieve&db=pubmed&dopt=Abstract&list_uids=947035

- **Acute dystonic reactions that fail to respond to diphenhydramine: think of PCP.**
  Author(s): Piecuch S, Thomas U, Shah BR.
  Source: The Journal of Emergency Medicine. 1999 May-June; 17(3): 527.
  http://www.ncbi.nlm.nih.gov/entrez/query.fcgi?cmd=Retrieve&db=pubmed&dopt=Abstract&list_uids=10338254

- **Acute intoxication with guaifenesin, diphenhydramine, and chlorpheniramine.**
  Author(s): Wogoman H, Steinberg M, Jenkins AJ.
  Source: The American Journal of Forensic Medicine and Pathology : Official Publication of the National Association of Medical Examiners. 1999 June; 20(2): 199-202.
  http://www.ncbi.nlm.nih.gov/entrez/query.fcgi?cmd=Retrieve&db=pubmed&dopt=Abstract&list_uids=10414664

- **Allergic and photoallergic dermatitis from diphenhydramine.**
  Author(s): Horio T.
  Source: Archives of Dermatology. 1976 August; 112(8): 1124-6.
  http://www.ncbi.nlm.nih.gov/entrez/query.fcgi?cmd=Retrieve&db=pubmed&dopt=Abstract&list_uids=952531

- **An electroencephalographic study on the tolerance of psychiatric and neurologic patients to the hypnotic effect of diphenhydramine.**
  Author(s): Okuma T, Kawahara R, Umezawa Y, Kashiwagi T.
  Source: Folia Psychiatr Neurol Jpn. 1973; 27(2): 85-104. No Abstract Available.
  http://www.ncbi.nlm.nih.gov/entrez/query.fcgi?cmd=Retrieve&db=pubmed&dopt=Abstract&list_uids=4741009

- **An experimental evaluation of dependence liability of methaqualone diphenhydramine (combination) and methaqualone in rats.**
  Author(s): Singh N, Nath R, Kulshrestha VK, Kohli RP.
  Source: Psychopharmacology. 1980 February; 67(2): 203-7.
  http://www.ncbi.nlm.nih.gov/entrez/query.fcgi?cmd=Retrieve&db=pubmed&dopt=Abstract&list_uids=6768095

- **An unusual vasculitis due to diphenhydramine. Cutaneous and central nervous system involvement.**
  Author(s): Davenport PM, Wilhelm RE.
  Source: Archives of Dermatology. 1965 November; 92(5): 577-80.
  http://www.ncbi.nlm.nih.gov/entrez/query.fcgi?cmd=Retrieve&db=pubmed&dopt=Abstract&list_uids=4221165

- **Anaphylactic reaction due to diphenhydramine.**
  Author(s): Barranco P, Lopez-Serrano MC, Moreno-Ancillo A.
  Source: Allergy. 1998 August; 53(8): 814.
  http://www.ncbi.nlm.nih.gov/entrez/query.fcgi?cmd=Retrieve&db=pubmed&dopt=Abstract&list_uids=9722235

- **Antiemetic control and prevention of side effects of anti-cancer therapy with lorazepam or diphenhydramine when used in combination with metoclopramide plus dexamethasone. A double-blind, randomized trial.**
  Author(s): Kris MG, Gralla RJ, Clark RA, Tyson LB, Groshen S.
  Source: Cancer. 1987 December 1; 60(11): 2816-22.
  http://www.ncbi.nlm.nih.gov/entrez/query.fcgi?cmd=Retrieve&db=pubmed&dopt=Abstract&list_uids=3315176

- **Antiemetic efficacy of droperidol or metoclopramide combined with dexamethasone and diphenhydramine. Randomized open parallel study.**
  Author(s): Aapro MS, Froidevaux P, Roth A, Alberto P.
  Source: Oncology. 1991; 48(2): 116-20.
  http://www.ncbi.nlm.nih.gov/entrez/query.fcgi?cmd=Retrieve&db=pubmed&dopt=Abstract&list_uids=1997933

- **Antiemetic efficacy of high-dose dexamethasone: randomized, double-blind, crossover study with a combination of dexamethasone, metoclopramide and diphenhydramine.**
  Author(s): al-Idrissi HY, Ibrahim EM, Abdullah KA, Ababtain WA, Boukhary HA, Macaulay HM.
  Source: British Journal of Cancer. 1988 March; 57(3): 308-12.
  http://www.ncbi.nlm.nih.gov/entrez/query.fcgi?cmd=Retrieve&db=pubmed&dopt=Abstract&list_uids=3281702

- **Antitussive activity of diphenhydramine in chronic cough.**
  Author(s): Lilienfield LS, Rose JC, Princiotto JV.
  Source: Clinical Pharmacology and Therapeutics. 1976 April; 19(4): 421-5.
  http://www.ncbi.nlm.nih.gov/entrez/query.fcgi?cmd=Retrieve&db=pubmed&dopt=Abstract&list_uids=773581

- **Antitussive effects of diphenhydramine on the citric acid aerosol-induced cough response in humans.**
  Author(s): Packman EW, Ciccone PE, Wilson J, Masurat T.
  Source: Int J Clin Pharmacol Ther Toxicol. 1991 June; 29(6): 218-22.
  http://www.ncbi.nlm.nih.gov/entrez/query.fcgi?cmd=Retrieve&db=pubmed&dopt=Abstract&list_uids=1869343

- **Association of diphenhydramine use with adverse effects in hospitalized older patients: possible confounders.**
  Author(s): Meuleman JR.
  Source: Archives of Internal Medicine. 2002 March 25; 162(6): 720-1.
  http://www.ncbi.nlm.nih.gov/entrez/query.fcgi?cmd=Retrieve&db=pubmed&dopt=Abstract&list_uids=11911733

- **Asynchronies of diphenhydramine plasma-performance relationships.**
  Author(s): Licko V, Thompson T, Barnett G.
  Source: Pharmacology, Biochemistry, and Behavior. 1986 August; 25(2): 365-70.
  http://www.ncbi.nlm.nih.gov/entrez/query.fcgi?cmd=Retrieve&db=pubmed&dopt=Abstract&list_uids=3763663

- **Beneficial effects of diphenhydramine in dystonia.**
  Author(s): Granana N, Ferrea M, Scorticati MC, Diaz S, Arrebola M, Torres L, Micheli F.
  Source: Medicina (B Aires). 1999; 59(1): 38-42.
  http://www.ncbi.nlm.nih.gov/entrez/query.fcgi?cmd=Retrieve&db=pubmed&dopt=Abstract&list_uids=10349117

- **Biphasic kinetics of quaternary ammonium glucuronide formation from amitriptyline and diphenhydramine in human liver microsomes.**
  Author(s): Breyer-Pfaff U, Fischer D, Winne D.
  Source: Drug Metabolism and Disposition: the Biological Fate of Chemicals. 1997 March; 25(3): 340-5.
  http://www.ncbi.nlm.nih.gov/entrez/query.fcgi?cmd=Retrieve&db=pubmed&dopt=Abstract&list_uids=9172952

- **Block of potassium currents in guinea pig ventricular myocytes and lengthening of cardiac repolarization in man by the histamine H1 receptor antagonist diphenhydramine.**
  Author(s): Khalifa M, Drolet B, Daleau P, Lefez C, Gilbert M, Plante S, O'Hara GE, Gleeton O, Hamelin BA, Turgeon J.
  Source: The Journal of Pharmacology and Experimental Therapeutics. 1999 February; 288(2): 858-65.
  http://www.ncbi.nlm.nih.gov/entrez/query.fcgi?cmd=Retrieve&db=pubmed&dopt=Abstract&list_uids=9918600

- **Central anticholinergic syndrome after ofloxacin overdose and therapeutic doses of diphenhydramine and chlormezanone.**
  Author(s): Koppel C, Hopfe T, Menzel J.
  Source: Journal of Toxicology. Clinical Toxicology. 1990; 28(2): 249-53.
  http://www.ncbi.nlm.nih.gov/entrez/query.fcgi?cmd=Retrieve&db=pubmed&dopt=Abstract&list_uids=2398523

- **Children's school performance is not impaired by short-term administration of diphenhydramine or loratadine.**
  Author(s): Bender BG, McCormick DR, Milgrom H.
  Source: The Journal of Pediatrics. 2001 May; 138(5): 656-60.
  http://www.ncbi.nlm.nih.gov/entrez/query.fcgi?cmd=Retrieve&db=pubmed&dopt=Abstract&list_uids=11343039

- **Clinical evaluation of diphenhydramine hydrochloride for the treatment of insomnia in psychiatric patients: a double-blind study.**
  Author(s): Kudo Y, Kurihara M.
  Source: Journal of Clinical Pharmacology. 1990 November; 30(11): 1041-8.
  http://www.ncbi.nlm.nih.gov/entrez/query.fcgi?cmd=Retrieve&db=pubmed&dopt=Abstract&list_uids=2243152

- **Clinical evaluation of Sedyn-A-forte, an analgesic injection containing analgin, diphenhydramine and diazepam.**
  Author(s): Albal MV, Chandorkar AG.
  Source: Indian J Ophthalmol. 1982 July; 30(4): 271-3. No Abstract Available.
  http://www.ncbi.nlm.nih.gov/entrez/query.fcgi?cmd=Retrieve&db=pubmed&dopt=Abstract&list_uids=7166403

- **Clinical symptomatology of diphenhydramine overdose: an evaluation of 136 cases in 1982 to 1985.**
  Author(s): Koppel C, Ibe K, Tenczer J.
  Source: Journal of Toxicology. Clinical Toxicology. 1987; 25(1-2): 53-70.
  http://www.ncbi.nlm.nih.gov/entrez/query.fcgi?cmd=Retrieve&db=pubmed&dopt=Abstract&list_uids=3586086

- **CNS effects of the antihistamines diphenhydramine and terfenadine (RMI 9918).**
  Author(s): Fink M, Irwin P.
  Source: Pharmakopsychiatr Neuropsychopharmakol. 1979 January; 12(1): 35-44.
  http://www.ncbi.nlm.nih.gov/entrez/query.fcgi?cmd=Retrieve&db=pubmed&dopt=Abstract&list_uids=33398

- **Cognitive and other adverse effects of diphenhydramine use in hospitalized older patients.**
  Author(s): Agostini JV, Leo-Summers LS, Inouye SK.
  Source: Archives of Internal Medicine. 2001 September 24; 161(17): 2091-7.
  http://www.ncbi.nlm.nih.gov/entrez/query.fcgi?cmd=Retrieve&db=pubmed&dopt=Abstract&list_uids=11570937

- **Combination metoclopramide and diphenhydramine short infusion for prevention of chemotherapy-induced emesis.**
  Author(s): Przepiorka D, Katlubeck A, Taylor D.
  Source: American Journal of Clinical Oncology : the Official Publication of the American Radium Society. 1990 April; 13(2): 180.
  http://www.ncbi.nlm.nih.gov/entrez/query.fcgi?cmd=Retrieve&db=pubmed&dopt=Abstract&list_uids=2316485

- **Comment: Rhabdomyolysis and acute renal failure following an ethanol and diphenhydramine overdose.**
  Author(s): Mycyk MB, Mazor SS.
  Source: The Annals of Pharmacotherapy. 2003 September; 37(9): 1345; Author Reply 1345-6.
  http://www.ncbi.nlm.nih.gov/entrez/query.fcgi?cmd=Retrieve&db=pubmed&dopt=Abstract&list_uids=12921526

- **Comparison of cimetidine and diphenhydramine in the treatment of acute urticaria.**
  Author(s): Moscati RM, Moore GP.
  Source: Annals of Emergency Medicine. 1990 January; 19(1): 12-5.
  http://www.ncbi.nlm.nih.gov/entrez/query.fcgi?cmd=Retrieve&db=pubmed&dopt=Abstract&list_uids=2404434

- **Comparison of effects of lidocaine hydrochloride, buffered lidocaine, diphenhydramine, and normal saline after intradermal injection.**
  Author(s): Xia Y, Chen E, Tibbits DL, Reilley TE, McSweeney TD.
  Source: Journal of Clinical Anesthesia. 2002 August; 14(5): 339-43.
  http://www.ncbi.nlm.nih.gov/entrez/query.fcgi?cmd=Retrieve&db=pubmed&dopt=Abstract&list_uids=12208437

- **Comparison of procedures for measuring the quaternary N-glucuronides of amitriptyline and diphenhydramine in human urine with and without hydrolysis.**
  Author(s): Fischer D, Breyer-Pfaff U.
  Source: The Journal of Pharmacy and Pharmacology. 1995 June; 47(6): 534-8.
  http://www.ncbi.nlm.nih.gov/entrez/query.fcgi?cmd=Retrieve&db=pubmed&dopt=Abstract&list_uids=7674140

- **Comparison of the efficacy and side-effects of ondansetron and metoclopramide-diphenhydramine administered to control nausea and vomiting in children treated with antineoplastic chemotherapy: a prospective randomized study.**
  Author(s): Koseoglu V, Kurekci AE, Sarici U, Atay AA, Ozcan O, Sorici U.
  Source: European Journal of Pediatrics. 1998 October; 157(10): 806-10. Erratum In: Eur J Pediatr 1999 February; 158(2): 168. Sorici U[corrected to Sarici U].
  http://www.ncbi.nlm.nih.gov/entrez/query.fcgi?cmd=Retrieve&db=pubmed&dopt=Abstract&list_uids=9809818

- **Compatibility of haloperidol and diphenhydramine in a hypodermic syringe.**
  Author(s): Ukhun IA.
  Source: The Annals of Pharmacotherapy. 1995 November; 29(11): 1168-9.
  http://www.ncbi.nlm.nih.gov/entrez/query.fcgi?cmd=Retrieve&db=pubmed&dopt=Abstract&list_uids=8573967

- **Complications of methaqualone-diphenhydramine (Mandrax R) abuse.**
  Author(s): Tennant FS.
  Source: The British Journal of Addiction to Alcohol and Other Drugs. 1973 December; 68(4): 327-30.
  http://www.ncbi.nlm.nih.gov/entrez/query.fcgi?cmd=Retrieve&db=pubmed&dopt=Abstract&list_uids=4528484

- **Consecutive dose-finding trials adding lorazepam to the combination of metoclopramide plus dexamethasone: improved subjective effectiveness over the combination of diphenhydramine plus metoclopramide plus dexamethasone.**
  Author(s): Kris MG, Gralla RJ, Clark RA, Tyson LB, Fiore JJ, Kelsen DP, Groshen S.
  Source: Cancer Treat Rep. 1985 November; 69(11): 1257-62.
  http://www.ncbi.nlm.nih.gov/entrez/query.fcgi?cmd=Retrieve&db=pubmed&dopt=Abstract&list_uids=3912039

- **Contact dermatitis caused by diphenhydramine hydrochloride.**
  Author(s): Coskey RJ.
  Source: Journal of the American Academy of Dermatology. 1983 February; 8(2): 204-6.
  http://www.ncbi.nlm.nih.gov/entrez/query.fcgi?cmd=Retrieve&db=pubmed&dopt=Abstract&list_uids=6219138

- **Correlation between plasma diphenhydramine level and sedative and antihistamine effects.**
  Author(s): Carruthers SG, Shoeman DW, Hignite CE, Azarnoff DL.
  Source: Clinical Pharmacology and Therapeutics. 1978 April; 23(4): 375-82.
  http://www.ncbi.nlm.nih.gov/entrez/query.fcgi?cmd=Retrieve&db=pubmed&dopt=Abstract&list_uids=24512

- **Determination of diphenhydramine in plasma by gas chromatography.**
  Author(s): Albert KS, Sakmar E, Morais JA, Hallmark MR, Wagner JG.
  Source: Res Commun Chem Pathol Pharmacol. 1974 January; 7(1): 95-103. No Abstract Available.
  http://www.ncbi.nlm.nih.gov/entrez/query.fcgi?cmd=Retrieve&db=pubmed&dopt=Abstract&list_uids=4149497

- **Determination of nanogram quantities of diphenhydramine and orphenadrine in human plasma using gas-liquid chromatography.**
  Author(s): Bilzer W, Gundert-Remy U.
  Source: European Journal of Clinical Pharmacology. 1973 December; 6(4): 268-70.
  http://www.ncbi.nlm.nih.gov/entrez/query.fcgi?cmd=Retrieve&db=pubmed&dopt=Abstract&list_uids=4777260

- **Differentiating the effects of centrally acting drugs on arousal and memory: an event-related potential study of scopolamine, lorazepam and diphenhydramine.**
  Author(s): Curran HV, Pooviboonsuk P, Dalton JA, Lader MH.
  Source: Psychopharmacology. 1998 January; 135(1): 27-36.
  http://www.ncbi.nlm.nih.gov/entrez/query.fcgi?cmd=Retrieve&db=pubmed&dopt=Abstract&list_uids=9489931

- **Diphenhydramine (Unisom), a central anticholinergic and antihistaminic: abuse with massive ingestion in a patient with schizophrenia.**
  Author(s): Barsoum A, Kolivakis TT, Margolese HC, Chouinard G.
  Source: Canadian Journal of Psychiatry. Revue Canadienne De Psychiatrie. 2000 November; 45(9): 846-7.
  http://www.ncbi.nlm.nih.gov/entrez/query.fcgi?cmd=Retrieve&db=pubmed&dopt=Abstract&list_uids=11143840

- **Diphenhydramine abuse and withdrawal.**
  Author(s): Glickman L.
  Source: Jama : the Journal of the American Medical Association. 1986 October 10; 256(14): 1894.
  http://www.ncbi.nlm.nih.gov/entrez/query.fcgi?cmd=Retrieve&db=pubmed&dopt=Abstract&list_uids=3761494

- **Diphenhydramine alters the disposition of venlafaxine through inhibition of CYP2D6 activity in humans.**
  Author(s): Lessard E, Yessine MA, Hamelin BA, Gauvin C, Labbe L, O'Hara G, LeBlanc J, Turgeon J.
  Source: Journal of Clinical Psychopharmacology. 2001 April; 21(2): 175-84.
  http://www.ncbi.nlm.nih.gov/entrez/query.fcgi?cmd=Retrieve&db=pubmed&dopt=Abstract&list_uids=11270914

- **Diphenhydramine and acute dystonia.**
  Author(s): Roila F, Donati D, Basurto C, Del Favero A.
  Source: Annals of Internal Medicine. 1989 July 1; 111(1): 92-3.
  http://www.ncbi.nlm.nih.gov/entrez/query.fcgi?cmd=Retrieve&db=pubmed&dopt=Abstract&list_uids=2735633

- **Diphenhydramine and Asians.**
  Author(s): Brown T.
  Source: Journal of the American Pharmaceutical Association (Washington,D.C. : 1996). 1996 October; Ns36(10): 563.
  http://www.ncbi.nlm.nih.gov/entrez/query.fcgi?cmd=Retrieve&db=pubmed&dopt=Abstract&list_uids=8908928

- **Diphenhydramine and the calcium carbimide-ethanol reaction: a placebo-controlled clinical study.**
  Author(s): Stowell A, Johnsen J, Ripel A, Morland J.
  Source: Clinical Pharmacology and Therapeutics. 1986 May; 39(5): 521-5.
  http://www.ncbi.nlm.nih.gov/entrez/query.fcgi?cmd=Retrieve&db=pubmed&dopt=Abstract&list_uids=3516510

- **Diphenhydramine as an analgesic adjuvant in refractory cancer pain.**
  Author(s): Santiago-Palma J, Fischberg D, Kornick C, Khjainova N, Gonzales G.
  Source: Journal of Pain and Symptom Management. 2001 August; 22(2): 699-703.
  http://www.ncbi.nlm.nih.gov/entrez/query.fcgi?cmd=Retrieve&db=pubmed&dopt=Abstract&list_uids=11495716

- **Diphenhydramine dependence.**
  Author(s): Cox D, Ahmed Z, McBride AJ.
  Source: Addiction (Abingdon, England). 2001 March; 96(3): 516-7. Review.
  http://www.ncbi.nlm.nih.gov/entrez/query.fcgi?cmd=Retrieve&db=pubmed&dopt=A
  bstract&list_uids=11310441

- **Diphenhydramine dependence: a need for awareness.**
  Author(s): de Nesnera AP.
  Source: The Journal of Clinical Psychiatry. 1996 March; 57(3): 136-7.
  http://www.ncbi.nlm.nih.gov/entrez/query.fcgi?cmd=Retrieve&db=pubmed&dopt=A
  bstract&list_uids=8617701

- **Diphenhydramine determination in human plasma by gas-liquid chromatography using nitrogen-phosphorus detection: application to single low-dose pharmacokinetic studies.**
  Author(s): Abernethy DR, Greenblatt DJ.
  Source: Journal of Pharmaceutical Sciences. 1983 August; 72(8): 941-3.
  http://www.ncbi.nlm.nih.gov/entrez/query.fcgi?cmd=Retrieve&db=pubmed&dopt=A
  bstract&list_uids=6620153

- **Diphenhydramine disposition in chronic liver disease.**
  Author(s): Meredith CG, Christian CD Jr, Johnson RF, Madhavan SV, Schenker S.
  Source: Clinical Pharmacology and Therapeutics. 1984 April; 35(4): 474-9.
  http://www.ncbi.nlm.nih.gov/entrez/query.fcgi?cmd=Retrieve&db=pubmed&dopt=A
  bstract&list_uids=6705445

- **Diphenhydramine disposition in the sheep maternal-placental-fetal unit: determinants of plasma drug concentrations in the mother and the fetus.**
  Author(s): Kumar S, Tonn GR, Riggs KW, Rurak DW.
  Source: Journal of Pharmaceutical Sciences. 1999 December; 88(12): 1259-65.
  http://www.ncbi.nlm.nih.gov/entrez/query.fcgi?cmd=Retrieve&db=pubmed&dopt=A
  bstract&list_uids=10585220

- **Diphenhydramine enhances the interaction of hypercapnic and hypoxic ventilatory drive.**
  Author(s): Alexander CM, Seifert HA, Blouin RT, Conard PF, Gross JB.
  Source: Anesthesiology. 1994 April; 80(4): 789-95.
  http://www.ncbi.nlm.nih.gov/entrez/query.fcgi?cmd=Retrieve&db=pubmed&dopt=A
  bstract&list_uids=8024132

- **Diphenhydramine for local anesthesia in "caine" sensitive patients. A case report.**
  Author(s): Munsey WF.
  Source: J Am Podiatry Assoc. 1966 January; 56(1): 25-6. No Abstract Available.
  http://www.ncbi.nlm.nih.gov/entrez/query.fcgi?cmd=Retrieve&db=pubmed&dopt=A
  bstract&list_uids=5903260

- **Diphenhydramine for nausea and vomiting related to cancer chemotherapy with cisplatin.**
  Author(s): Tsavaris NB.
  Source: Journal of Pain and Symptom Management. 1992 November; 7(8): 440-2.
  http://www.ncbi.nlm.nih.gov/entrez/query.fcgi?cmd=Retrieve&db=pubmed&dopt=Abstract&list_uids=1287105

- **Diphenhydramine for nausea and vomiting related to cancer chemotherapy with cisplatin.**
  Author(s): Tsavaris N, Zamanis N, Zinelis A, Tsoutsos E, Mylonakis N, Bacoyannis C, Valilis P, Sarafidou M, Kosmidis P.
  Source: Journal of Pain and Symptom Management. 1991 November; 6(8): 461-5.
  http://www.ncbi.nlm.nih.gov/entrez/query.fcgi?cmd=Retrieve&db=pubmed&dopt=Abstract&list_uids=1955741

- **Diphenhydramine for the prevention of akathisia induced by prochlorperazine: a randomized, controlled trial.**
  Author(s): Vinson DR, Drotts DL.
  Source: Annals of Emergency Medicine. 2001 February; 37(2): 125-31.
  http://www.ncbi.nlm.nih.gov/entrez/query.fcgi?cmd=Retrieve&db=pubmed&dopt=Abstract&list_uids=11174228

- **Diphenhydramine gargling may slow the healing of oral lesions of pemphigus vulgaris.**
  Author(s): Namazi MR.
  Source: J Drugs Dermatol. 2004 January-February; 3(1): 12. No Abstract Available.
  http://www.ncbi.nlm.nih.gov/entrez/query.fcgi?cmd=Retrieve&db=pubmed&dopt=Abstract&list_uids=14964741

- **Diphenhydramine hydrochloride as a local anesthetic. A case report.**
  Author(s): Howard K, Conrad T, Heiser J, Manzi JA.
  Source: J Am Podiatry Assoc. 1984 May; 74(5): 240-2. No Abstract Available.
  http://www.ncbi.nlm.nih.gov/entrez/query.fcgi?cmd=Retrieve&db=pubmed&dopt=Abstract&list_uids=6725849

- **Diphenhydramine hydrochloride helps symptoms of ciguatera fish poisoning.**
  Author(s): Savaloja J.
  Source: Journal of Emergency Nursing: Jen : Official Publication of the Emergency Department Nurses Association. 1996 October; 22(5): 373.
  http://www.ncbi.nlm.nih.gov/entrez/query.fcgi?cmd=Retrieve&db=pubmed&dopt=Abstract&list_uids=8997960

- **Diphenhydramine hydrochloride in premedication for cardiac catheterization.**
  Author(s): Akdikmen SA, Rosenthal R, Landmesser CM.
  Source: Anesthesia and Analgesia. 1966 May-June; 45(3): 293-7.
  http://www.ncbi.nlm.nih.gov/entrez/query.fcgi?cmd=Retrieve&db=pubmed&dopt=Abstract&list_uids=5949158

- **Diphenhydramine hydrochloride intoxication.**
  Author(s): Hestand HE, Teske DW.
  Source: The Journal of Pediatrics. 1977 June; 90(6): 1017-8.
  http://www.ncbi.nlm.nih.gov/entrez/query.fcgi?cmd=Retrieve&db=pubmed&dopt=Abstract&list_uids=859051

- **Diphenhydramine in insomniac family practice patients: a double-blind study.**
  Author(s): Rickels K, Morris RJ, Newman H, Rosenfeld H, Schiller H, Weinstock R.
  Source: Journal of Clinical Pharmacology. 1983 May-June; 23(5-6): 234-42.
  http://www.ncbi.nlm.nih.gov/entrez/query.fcgi?cmd=Retrieve&db=pubmed&dopt=Abstract&list_uids=6348106

- **Diphenhydramine in Orientals and Caucasians.**
  Author(s): Spector R, Choudhury AK, Chiang CK, Goldberg MJ, Ghoneim MM.
  Source: Clinical Pharmacology and Therapeutics. 1980 August; 28(2): 229-34.
  http://www.ncbi.nlm.nih.gov/entrez/query.fcgi?cmd=Retrieve&db=pubmed&dopt=Abstract&list_uids=7398190

- **Diphenhydramine in the differential diagnosis of neuroleptic-induced oral-facial dyskinesia.**
  Author(s): Beitman BD.
  Source: The American Journal of Psychiatry. 1977 June; 134(6): 695-6.
  http://www.ncbi.nlm.nih.gov/entrez/query.fcgi?cmd=Retrieve&db=pubmed&dopt=Abstract&list_uids=869040

- **Diphenhydramine interferes with determination of phencyclidine by gas-liquid chromatography.**
  Author(s): Ragan FA Jr, Samuels MS, Hite SA, Ory R.
  Source: Clinical Chemistry. 1980 May; 26(6): 785-6.
  http://www.ncbi.nlm.nih.gov/entrez/query.fcgi?cmd=Retrieve&db=pubmed&dopt=Abstract&list_uids=7371165

- **Diphenhydramine is effective in the treatment of idiopathic dystonia.**
  Author(s): Truong DD, Sandroni P, van den Noort S, Matsumoto RR.
  Source: Archives of Neurology. 1995 April; 52(4): 405-7.
  http://www.ncbi.nlm.nih.gov/entrez/query.fcgi?cmd=Retrieve&db=pubmed&dopt=Abstract&list_uids=7710376

- **Diphenhydramine kinetics following intravenous, oral, and sublingual dimenhydrinate administration.**
  Author(s): Scavone JM, Luna BG, Harmatz JS, von Moltke L, Greenblatt DJ.
  Source: Biopharmaceutics & Drug Disposition. 1990 April; 11(3): 185-9.
  http://www.ncbi.nlm.nih.gov/entrez/query.fcgi?cmd=Retrieve&db=pubmed&dopt=Abstract&list_uids=2328304

- **Diphenhydramine overdose during pregnancy: lessons from the past.**
  Author(s): Brost BC, Scardo JA, Newman RB.
  Source: American Journal of Obstetrics and Gynecology. 1996 November; 175(5): 1376-7.
  http://www.ncbi.nlm.nih.gov/entrez/query.fcgi?cmd=Retrieve&db=pubmed&dopt=Abstract&list_uids=8942519

- **Diphenhydramine photoallergy.**
  Author(s): Emmett EA.
  Source: Archives of Dermatology. 1974 August; 110(2): 249-52.
  http://www.ncbi.nlm.nih.gov/entrez/query.fcgi?cmd=Retrieve&db=pubmed&dopt=A
  bstract&list_uids=4277438

- **Diphenhydramine prevents the haemodynamic changes of cimetidine in ICU patients.**
  Author(s): Omote K, Namiki A, Iwasaki H, Ujike Y.
  Source: Canadian Journal of Anaesthesia = Journal Canadien D'anesthesie. 1991 March;
  38(2): 210-2.
  http://www.ncbi.nlm.nih.gov/entrez/query.fcgi?cmd=Retrieve&db=pubmed&dopt=A
  bstract&list_uids=2021990

- **Diphenhydramine provides relief of cyclophosphamide-related symptoms.**
  Author(s): Purl S, Johnson L, Hanauer S, Schroeder L, Proeschel C, Alberts J.
  Source: Oncology Nursing Forum. 1996 April; 23(3): 542.
  http://www.ncbi.nlm.nih.gov/entrez/query.fcgi?cmd=Retrieve&db=pubmed&dopt=A
  bstract&list_uids=8801517

- **Diphenhydramine reversal of vancomycin-induced hypotension.**
  Author(s): Lyon GD, Bruce DL.
  Source: Anesthesia and Analgesia. 1988 November; 67(11): 1109-10.
  http://www.ncbi.nlm.nih.gov/entrez/query.fcgi?cmd=Retrieve&db=pubmed&dopt=A
  bstract&list_uids=3189903

- **Diphenhydramine toxicity from combined oral and topical use.**
  Author(s): Schunk JE, Svendsen D.
  Source: Am J Dis Child. 1988 October; 142(10): 1020-1. No Abstract Available.
  http://www.ncbi.nlm.nih.gov/entrez/query.fcgi?cmd=Retrieve&db=pubmed&dopt=A
  bstract&list_uids=3177290

- **Diphenhydramine toxicity in a child with varicella. A case report.**
  Author(s): McGann KP, Pribanich S, Graham JA, Browning DG.
  Source: The Journal of Family Practice. 1992 August; 35(2): 210, 213-4.
  http://www.ncbi.nlm.nih.gov/entrez/query.fcgi?cmd=Retrieve&db=pubmed&dopt=A
  bstract&list_uids=1645115

- **Diphenhydramine toxicity in a newborn: a case report.**
  Author(s): Miller AA.
  Source: Journal of Perinatology : Official Journal of the California Perinatal Association.
  2000 September; 20(6): 390-1.
  http://www.ncbi.nlm.nih.gov/entrez/query.fcgi?cmd=Retrieve&db=pubmed&dopt=A
  bstract&list_uids=11002881

- **Diphenhydramine toxicity in three children with varicella-zoster infection.**
  Author(s): Chan CY, Wallander KA.
  Source: Dicp. 1991 February; 25(2): 130-2. Review.
  http://www.ncbi.nlm.nih.gov/entrez/query.fcgi?cmd=Retrieve&db=pubmed&dopt=Abstract&list_uids=2058184

- **Diphenhydramine toxicity mimicking varicella encephalitis.**
  Author(s): Tomlinson G, Helfaer M, Wiedermann BL.
  Source: The Pediatric Infectious Disease Journal. 1987 February; 6(2): 220-1.
  http://www.ncbi.nlm.nih.gov/entrez/query.fcgi?cmd=Retrieve&db=pubmed&dopt=Abstract&list_uids=3562147

- **Diphenhydramine toxicity: comparisons of postmortem findings in diphenhydramine-, cocaine-, and heroin-related deaths.**
  Author(s): Karch SB.
  Source: The American Journal of Forensic Medicine and Pathology : Official Publication of the National Association of Medical Examiners. 1998 June; 19(2): 143-7.
  http://www.ncbi.nlm.nih.gov/entrez/query.fcgi?cmd=Retrieve&db=pubmed&dopt=Abstract&list_uids=9662109

- **Diphenhydramine transport by pH-dependent tertiary amine transport system in Caco-2 cells.**
  Author(s): Mizuuchi H, Katsura T, Ashida K, Hashimoto Y, Inui K.
  Source: American Journal of Physiology. Gastrointestinal and Liver Physiology. 2000 April; 278(4): G563-9.
  http://www.ncbi.nlm.nih.gov/entrez/query.fcgi?cmd=Retrieve&db=pubmed&dopt=Abstract&list_uids=10762610

- **Diphenhydramine.**
  Author(s): Garnett WR.
  Source: Am Pharm. 1986 February; Ns26(2): 35-40. No Abstract Available.
  http://www.ncbi.nlm.nih.gov/entrez/query.fcgi?cmd=Retrieve&db=pubmed&dopt=Abstract&list_uids=3962845

- **Diphenhydramine/vancomycin admixture for infusion phlebitis.**
  Author(s): Fisher CH, Fiorilli MG, Maradiaga CM.
  Source: The Annals of Pharmacotherapy. 1996 December; 30(12): 1495.
  http://www.ncbi.nlm.nih.gov/entrez/query.fcgi?cmd=Retrieve&db=pubmed&dopt=Abstract&list_uids=8968464

- **Diphenhydramine: a forgotten allergen?**
  Author(s): Heine A.
  Source: Contact Dermatitis. 1996 November; 35(5): 311-2.
  http://www.ncbi.nlm.nih.gov/entrez/query.fcgi?cmd=Retrieve&db=pubmed&dopt=Abstract&list_uids=9007386

- **Diphenhydramine: kinetics and psychomotor effects in elderly women.**
  Author(s): Berlinger WG, Goldberg MJ, Spector R, Chiang CK, Ghoneim M.
  Source: Clinical Pharmacology and Therapeutics. 1982 September; 32(3): 387-91.
  http://www.ncbi.nlm.nih.gov/entrez/query.fcgi?cmd=Retrieve&db=pubmed&dopt=Abstract&list_uids=7049503

- **Diphenhydramine: pharmacokinetics and pharmacodynamics in elderly adults, young adults, and children.**
  Author(s): Simons KJ, Watson WT, Martin TJ, Chen XY, Simons FE.
  Source: Journal of Clinical Pharmacology. 1990 July; 30(7): 665-71.
  http://www.ncbi.nlm.nih.gov/entrez/query.fcgi?cmd=Retrieve&db=pubmed&dopt=Abstract&list_uids=2391399

- **Diphenhydramine-induced acute dystonia.**
  Author(s): Etzel JV.
  Source: Pharmacotherapy. 1994 July-August; 14(4): 492-6.
  http://www.ncbi.nlm.nih.gov/entrez/query.fcgi?cmd=Retrieve&db=pubmed&dopt=Abstract&list_uids=7937288

- **Diphenhydramine-induced delirium in elderly hospitalized patients with mild dementia.**
  Author(s): Tejera CA, Saravay SM, Goldman E, Gluck L.
  Source: Psychosomatics. 1994 July-August; 35(4): 399-402.
  http://www.ncbi.nlm.nih.gov/entrez/query.fcgi?cmd=Retrieve&db=pubmed&dopt=Abstract&list_uids=8084991

- **Diphenhydramine-induced dystonia.**
  Author(s): Santora J, Rozek S, Samie MR.
  Source: Clin Pharm. 1989 July; 8(7): 471. No Abstract Available.
  http://www.ncbi.nlm.nih.gov/entrez/query.fcgi?cmd=Retrieve&db=pubmed&dopt=Abstract&list_uids=2752695

- **Diphenhydramine-induced psychosis with therapeutic doses.**
  Author(s): Sexton JD, Pronchik DJ.
  Source: The American Journal of Emergency Medicine. 1997 September; 15(5): 548-9.
  http://www.ncbi.nlm.nih.gov/entrez/query.fcgi?cmd=Retrieve&db=pubmed&dopt=Abstract&list_uids=9270406

- **Diphenhydramine-induced toxic psychosis.**
  Author(s): Jones J, Dougherty J, Cannon L.
  Source: The American Journal of Emergency Medicine. 1986 July; 4(4): 369-71.
  http://www.ncbi.nlm.nih.gov/entrez/query.fcgi?cmd=Retrieve&db=pubmed&dopt=Abstract&list_uids=3718632

- **Diphenhydramine-induced wide complex dysrhythmia responds to treatment with sodium bicarbonate.**
  Author(s): Sharma AN, Hexdall AH, Chang EK, Nelson LS, Hoffman RS.
  Source: The American Journal of Emergency Medicine. 2003 May; 21(3): 212-5.
  http://www.ncbi.nlm.nih.gov/entrez/query.fcgi?cmd=Retrieve&db=pubmed&dopt=Abstract&list_uids=12811715

- **Dose-dependent toxicity of diphenhydramine overdose.**
Author(s): Radovanovic D, Meier PJ, Guirguis M, Lorent JP, Kupferschmidt H.
Source: Human & Experimental Toxicology. 2000 September; 19(9): 489-95.
http://www.ncbi.nlm.nih.gov/entrez/query.fcgi?cmd=Retrieve&db=pubmed&dopt=A
bstract&list_uids=11204550

- **Double-blind crossover study comparing doxepin with diphenhydramine for the treatment of chronic urticaria.**
Author(s): Greene SL, Reed CE, Schroeter AL.
Source: Journal of the American Academy of Dermatology. 1985 April; 12(4): 669-75.
http://www.ncbi.nlm.nih.gov/entrez/query.fcgi?cmd=Retrieve&db=pubmed&dopt=A
bstract&list_uids=3886724

- **Double-blinded comparison of diphenhydramine versus lidocaine as a local anesthetic.**
Author(s): Dire DJ, Hogan DE.
Source: Annals of Emergency Medicine. 1993 September; 22(9): 1419-22.
http://www.ncbi.nlm.nih.gov/entrez/query.fcgi?cmd=Retrieve&db=pubmed&dopt=A
bstract&list_uids=8363115

- **Doxylamine and diphenhydramine pharmacokinetics in women on low-dose estrogen oral contraceptives.**
Author(s): Luna BG, Scavone JM, Greenblatt DJ.
Source: Journal of Clinical Pharmacology. 1989 March; 29(3): 257-60.
http://www.ncbi.nlm.nih.gov/entrez/query.fcgi?cmd=Retrieve&db=pubmed&dopt=A
bstract&list_uids=2723113

- **Driving ability after acute and sub-chronic administration of levocetirizine and diphenhydramine: a randomized, double-blind, placebo-controlled trial.**
Author(s): Verster JC, de Weert AM, Bijtjes SI, Aarab M, van Oosterwijck AW, Eijken EJ, Verbaten MN, Volkerts ER.
Source: Psychopharmacology. 2003 August; 169(1): 84-90. Epub 2003 April 30.
http://www.ncbi.nlm.nih.gov/entrez/query.fcgi?cmd=Retrieve&db=pubmed&dopt=A
bstract&list_uids=12721777

- **Droperidol and diphenhydramine in the management of hyperemesis gravidarum.**
Author(s): Nageotte MP, Briggs GG, Towers CV, Asrat T.
Source: American Journal of Obstetrics and Gynecology. 1996 June; 174(6): 1801-5; Discussion 1805-6.
http://www.ncbi.nlm.nih.gov/entrez/query.fcgi?cmd=Retrieve&db=pubmed&dopt=A
bstract&list_uids=8678143

- **Drug-induced acute dystonic reactions in children. Alternatives to diphenhydramine therapy.**
Author(s): Dahiya U, Noronha P.
Source: Postgraduate Medicine. 1984 April; 75(5): 286-7, 290.
http://www.ncbi.nlm.nih.gov/entrez/query.fcgi?cmd=Retrieve&db=pubmed&dopt=A
bstract&list_uids=6143309

- **Eczematous eruption from oral diphenhydramine.**
  Author(s): Lawrence CM, Byrne JP.
  Source: Contact Dermatitis. 1981 September; 7(5): 276-7.
  http://www.ncbi.nlm.nih.gov/entrez/query.fcgi?cmd=Retrieve&db=pubmed&dopt=A
  bstract&list_uids=7307489

- **EEG activation of 3 Hz spike and wave complexes, especially activation with diphenhydramine (benadryl).**
  Author(s): Kitagawa T, Takahashi K.
  Source: Folia Psychiatr Neurol Jpn. 1980; 34(3): 327-8. No Abstract Available.
  http://www.ncbi.nlm.nih.gov/entrez/query.fcgi?cmd=Retrieve&db=pubmed&dopt=A
  bstract&list_uids=7216027

- **EEG and behavioral effects of drug therapy in children. Chlorpromazine and diphenhydramine.**
  Author(s): Korein J, Fish B, Shapiro T, Gerner EW, Levidow L.
  Source: Archives of General Psychiatry. 1971 June; 24(6): 552-63.
  http://www.ncbi.nlm.nih.gov/entrez/query.fcgi?cmd=Retrieve&db=pubmed&dopt=A
  bstract&list_uids=4931044

- **Effect of diphenhydramine on subjective sleep parameters and on motor activity during bedtime.**
  Author(s): Borbely AA, Youmbi-Balderer G.
  Source: Int J Clin Pharmacol Ther Toxicol. 1988 August; 26(8): 392-6.
  http://www.ncbi.nlm.nih.gov/entrez/query.fcgi?cmd=Retrieve&db=pubmed&dopt=A
  bstract&list_uids=3220614

- **Effects of caffeine or diphenhydramine on visual vigilance.**
  Author(s): Fine BJ, Kobrick JL, Lieberman HR, Marlowe B, Riley RH, Tharion WJ.
  Source: Psychopharmacology. 1994 March; 114(2): 233-8.
  http://www.ncbi.nlm.nih.gov/entrez/query.fcgi?cmd=Retrieve&db=pubmed&dopt=A
  bstract&list_uids=7838913

- **Effects of diphenhydramine and alcohol on skills performance.**
  Author(s): Burns M, Moskowitz H.
  Source: European Journal of Clinical Pharmacology. 1980 April; 17(4): 259-66.
  http://www.ncbi.nlm.nih.gov/entrez/query.fcgi?cmd=Retrieve&db=pubmed&dopt=A
  bstract&list_uids=6995128

- **Effects of diphenhydramine on human eye movements.**
  Author(s): Hopfenbeck JR, Cowley DS, Radant A, Greenblatt DJ, Roy-Byrne PP.
  Source: Psychopharmacology. 1995 April; 118(3): 280-6.
  http://www.ncbi.nlm.nih.gov/entrez/query.fcgi?cmd=Retrieve&db=pubmed&dopt=A
  bstract&list_uids=7617820

- **Effects of diphenhydramine on immunoassays of phencyclidine in urine.**
  Author(s): Levine BS, Smith ML.
  Source: Clinical Chemistry. 1990 June; 36(6): 1258.
  http://www.ncbi.nlm.nih.gov/entrez/query.fcgi?cmd=Retrieve&db=pubmed&dopt=A
  bstract&list_uids=2357810

- **Effects of ethanol, diphenhydramine, and triazolam after a nap.**
  Author(s): Roehrs T, Claiborue D, Knox M, Roth T.
  Source: Neuropsychopharmacology : Official Publication of the American College of Neuropsychopharmacology. 1993 November; 9(3): 239-45.
  http://www.ncbi.nlm.nih.gov/entrez/query.fcgi?cmd=Retrieve&db=pubmed&dopt=Abstract&list_uids=8280348

- **Effects of fexofenadine, diphenhydramine, and alcohol on driving performance. A randomized, placebo-controlled trial in the Iowa driving simulator.**
  Author(s): Weiler JM, Bloomfield JR, Woodworth GG, Grant AR, Layton TA, Brown TL, McKenzie DR, Baker TW, Watson GS.
  Source: Annals of Internal Medicine. 2000 March 7; 132(5): 354-63.
  http://www.ncbi.nlm.nih.gov/entrez/query.fcgi?cmd=Retrieve&db=pubmed&dopt=Abstract&list_uids=10691585

- **Effects of fexofenadine, diphenhydramine, and placebo on performance of the test of variables of attention (TOVA).**
  Author(s): Mansfield L, Mendoza C, Flores J, Meeves SG.
  Source: Annals of Allergy, Asthma & Immunology : Official Publication of the American College of Allergy, Asthma, & Immunology. 2003 May; 90(5): 554-9. Erratum In: Ann Allergy Asthma Immunol. 2003 August; 91(2): 167.
  http://www.ncbi.nlm.nih.gov/entrez/query.fcgi?cmd=Retrieve&db=pubmed&dopt=Abstract&list_uids=12775138

- **Effects of semprex-D and diphenhydramine on learning in young adults with seasonal allergic rhinitis.**
  Author(s): Vuurman EF, van Veggel LM, Sanders RL, Muntjewerff ND, O'Hanlon, JF.
  Source: Annals of Allergy, Asthma & Immunology : Official Publication of the American College of Allergy, Asthma, & Immunology. 1996 March; 76(3): 247-52.
  http://www.ncbi.nlm.nih.gov/entrez/query.fcgi?cmd=Retrieve&db=pubmed&dopt=Abstract&list_uids=8634878

- **Effects of terfenadine and diphenhydramine alone or in combination with diazepam or alcohol on psychomotor performance and subjective feelings.**
  Author(s): Moser L, Huther KJ, Koch-Weser J, Lundt PV.
  Source: European Journal of Clinical Pharmacology. 1978 December 18; 14(6): 417-23.
  http://www.ncbi.nlm.nih.gov/entrez/query.fcgi?cmd=Retrieve&db=pubmed&dopt=Abstract&list_uids=33053

- **Effects of terfenadine and diphenhydramine on the CYP2D6 activity in healthy volunteers.**
  Author(s): Kortunay S, Bozkurt A, Basci NE, Kayaalp SO.
  Source: Eur J Drug Metab Pharmacokinet. 2002 July-September; 27(3): 171-4.
  http://www.ncbi.nlm.nih.gov/entrez/query.fcgi?cmd=Retrieve&db=pubmed&dopt=Abstract&list_uids=12365197

- **Effects of terfenadine, diphenhydramine, and placebo on skills performance.**
  Author(s): Moskowitz H, Burns M.
  Source: Cutis; Cutaneous Medicine for the Practitioner. 1988 October 27; 42(4A): 14-8.
  http://www.ncbi.nlm.nih.gov/entrez/query.fcgi?cmd=Retrieve&db=pubmed&dopt=A
  bstract&list_uids=2903812

- **Efficacy of diphenhydramine hydrochloride for local anesthesia before oral surgery.**
  Author(s): Gallo WJ, Ellis E 3rd.
  Source: The Journal of the American Dental Association. 1987 August; 115(2): 263-6.
  http://www.ncbi.nlm.nih.gov/entrez/query.fcgi?cmd=Retrieve&db=pubmed&dopt=A
  bstract&list_uids=3476650

- **Electrocardiographic findings in patients with diphenhydramine overdose.**
  Author(s): Zareba W, Moss AJ, Rosero SZ, Hajj-Ali R, Konecki J, Andrews M.
  Source: The American Journal of Cardiology. 1997 November 1; 80(9): 1168-73.
  http://www.ncbi.nlm.nih.gov/entrez/query.fcgi?cmd=Retrieve&db=pubmed&dopt=A
  bstract&list_uids=9359544

- **Eosinophilic peritonitis in CAPD: treatment with prednisone and diphenhydramine.**
  Author(s): Thakur SS, Unikowsky B, Prichard S.
  Source: Perit Dial Int. 1997 July-August; 17(4): 402-3. No Abstract Available.
  http://www.ncbi.nlm.nih.gov/entrez/query.fcgi?cmd=Retrieve&db=pubmed&dopt=A
  bstract&list_uids=9284473

- **Evaluation of a combination antiemetic regimen including iv high-dose metoclopramide, dexamethasone, and diphenhydramine in cisplatin-based chemotherapy regimens.**
  Author(s): Rosell R, Abad-Esteve A, Ribas-Mundo M, Moreno I.
  Source: Cancer Treat Rep. 1985 July-August; 69(7-8): 909-10. No Abstract Available.
  http://www.ncbi.nlm.nih.gov/entrez/query.fcgi?cmd=Retrieve&db=pubmed&dopt=A
  bstract&list_uids=4040428

- **Evaluation of temazepam and diphenhydramine as hypnotics in a nursing-home population.**
  Author(s): Meuleman JR, Nelson RC, Clark RL Jr.
  Source: Drug Intell Clin Pharm. 1987 September; 21(9): 716-20.
  http://www.ncbi.nlm.nih.gov/entrez/query.fcgi?cmd=Retrieve&db=pubmed&dopt=A
  bstract&list_uids=2888637

- **Fatal adult respiratory distress syndrome after diphenhydramine toxicity in a child: a case report.**
  Author(s): Lindsay CA, Williams GD, Levin DL.
  Source: Critical Care Medicine. 1995 April; 23(4): 777-81.
  http://www.ncbi.nlm.nih.gov/entrez/query.fcgi?cmd=Retrieve&db=pubmed&dopt=A
  bstract&list_uids=7712771

- **Fatal anaphylactic shock to hyoscine and diphenhydramine.**
  Author(s): Watanabe T, Funayama M, Morita M.
  Source: Journal of Toxicology. Clinical Toxicology. 1994; 32(5): 593-4.
  http://www.ncbi.nlm.nih.gov/entrez/query.fcgi?cmd=Retrieve&db=pubmed&dopt=Abstract&list_uids=7932920

- **Fatal anaphylactic shock to hyoscine and diphenhydramine: a doubtful diagnosis.**
  Author(s): Manhart AR, Egwiekhor OA, Jahns BE, Rynn KO.
  Source: Journal of Toxicology. Clinical Toxicology. 1995; 33(2): 189-91.
  http://www.ncbi.nlm.nih.gov/entrez/query.fcgi?cmd=Retrieve&db=pubmed&dopt=Abstract&list_uids=7897761

- **Fatal diphenhydramine intoxication in infants.**
  Author(s): Baker AM, Johnson DG, Levisky JA, Hearn WL, Moore KA, Levine B, Nelson SJ.
  Source: J Forensic Sci. 2003 March; 48(2): 425-8.
  http://www.ncbi.nlm.nih.gov/entrez/query.fcgi?cmd=Retrieve&db=pubmed&dopt=Abstract&list_uids=12665005

- **Fatal poisoning with methaqualone and diphenhydramine.**
  Author(s): Sanderson JH, Cowdell RH, Higgins G.
  Source: Lancet. 1966 October 8; 2(7467): 803-4.
  http://www.ncbi.nlm.nih.gov/entrez/query.fcgi?cmd=Retrieve&db=pubmed&dopt=Abstract&list_uids=4162340

- **Filamentary keratitis associated with diphenhydramine hydrochloride (Benadryl).**
  Author(s): Seedor JA, Lamberts D, Bergmann RB, Perry HD.
  Source: American Journal of Ophthalmology. 1986 March 15; 101(3): 376-7.
  http://www.ncbi.nlm.nih.gov/entrez/query.fcgi?cmd=Retrieve&db=pubmed&dopt=Abstract&list_uids=3953733

- **Fixed drug eruption caused by diphenhydramine.**
  Author(s): Dwyer CM, Dick D.
  Source: Journal of the American Academy of Dermatology. 1993 September; 29(3): 496-7.
  http://www.ncbi.nlm.nih.gov/entrez/query.fcgi?cmd=Retrieve&db=pubmed&dopt=Abstract&list_uids=8349874

- **Further studies on the mechanism of human histamine-induced asthma: the effect of an aerosolized H1 receptor antagonist (diphenhydramine).**
  Author(s): Casterline CL, Evans R.
  Source: The Journal of Allergy and Clinical Immunology. 1977 June; 59(6): 420-4.
  http://www.ncbi.nlm.nih.gov/entrez/query.fcgi?cmd=Retrieve&db=pubmed&dopt=Abstract&list_uids=16944

- **High-performance liquid chromatography method for the determination of diphenhydramine in human plasma.**
  Author(s): Selinger K, Prevost J, Hill HM.
  Source: Journal of Chromatography. 1990 April 6; 526(2): 597-602.
  http://www.ncbi.nlm.nih.gov/entrez/query.fcgi?cmd=Retrieve&db=pubmed&dopt=Abstract&list_uids=2362001

- **Hypnotic activity of diphenhydramine, methapyrilene, and placebo.**
  Author(s): Sunshine A, Zighelboim I, Laska E.
  Source: Journal of Clinical Pharmacology. 1978 August-September; 18(8-9): 425-31.
  http://www.ncbi.nlm.nih.gov/entrez/query.fcgi?cmd=Retrieve&db=pubmed&dopt=Abstract&list_uids=357456

- **Hypnotic efficacy of diphenhydramine, methapyrilene, and pentobarbital.**
  Author(s): Teutsch G, Mahler DL, Brown CR, Forrest WH Jr, James KE, Brown BW.
  Source: Clinical Pharmacology and Therapeutics. 1975 February; 17(2): 195-201.
  http://www.ncbi.nlm.nih.gov/entrez/query.fcgi?cmd=Retrieve&db=pubmed&dopt=Abstract&list_uids=1091393

- **Identification of drug-related cognitive impairment in older individuals. Challenge studies with diphenhydramine.**
  Author(s): Sands L, Katz IR, DiFilippo S, D'Angelo K, Boyce A, Cooper T.
  Source: The American Journal of Geriatric Psychiatry : Official Journal of the American Association for Geriatric Psychiatry. 1997 Spring; 5(2): 156-66.
  http://www.ncbi.nlm.nih.gov/entrez/query.fcgi?cmd=Retrieve&db=pubmed&dopt=Abstract&list_uids=9106379

- **Impairment of hemostasis in patients with severe hemophilia. Failure of diphenhydramine, chlorpromazine, and guaifenesin.**
  Author(s): Buchanan GR, Handin RI.
  Source: Jama : the Journal of the American Medical Association. 1978 November 10; 240(20): 2173-4.
  http://www.ncbi.nlm.nih.gov/entrez/query.fcgi?cmd=Retrieve&db=pubmed&dopt=Abstract&list_uids=702728

- **Improved control of cisplatin-induced emesis with high-dose metoclopramide and with combinations of metoclopramide, dexamethasone, and diphenhydramine. Results of consecutive trials in 255 patients.**
  Author(s): Kris MG, Gralla RJ, Tyson LB, Clark RA, Kelsen DP, Reilly LK, Groshen S, Bosl GJ, Kalman LA.
  Source: Cancer. 1985 February 1; 55(3): 527-34.
  http://www.ncbi.nlm.nih.gov/entrez/query.fcgi?cmd=Retrieve&db=pubmed&dopt=Abstract&list_uids=3880660

- **Inappropriateness of the association of diphenhydramine with diethylcarbamazine for the treatment of lymphatic filariasis.**
  Author(s): Dreyer G, de Andrade L.
  Source: J Trop Med Hyg. 1989 February; 92(1): 32-4.
  http://www.ncbi.nlm.nih.gov/entrez/query.fcgi?cmd=Retrieve&db=pubmed&dopt=Abstract&list_uids=2645415

- **Incompatibility of diphenhydramine hydrochloride (Benadryl) with meglumine iodipamide (Cholografin).**
  Author(s): Stevens JS.
  Source: Radiology. 1975 October; 117(1): 224-5.
  http://www.ncbi.nlm.nih.gov/entrez/query.fcgi?cmd=Retrieve&db=pubmed&dopt=Abstract&list_uids=1162066

- **Increased risk of serious injury following an initial prescription for diphenhydramine.**
  Author(s): Finkle WD, Adams JL, Greenland S, Melmon KL.
  Source: Annals of Allergy, Asthma & Immunology : Official Publication of the American College of Allergy, Asthma, & Immunology. 2002 September; 89(3): 244-50.
  http://www.ncbi.nlm.nih.gov/entrez/query.fcgi?cmd=Retrieve&db=pubmed&dopt=Abstract&list_uids=12269643

- **Induction of the six c/sec spike and wave by diphenhydramine hydrochloride in healthy male adults.**
  Author(s): Hosokawa K, Hirata J, Kugoh T, Otsuki S.
  Source: Folia Psychiatr Neurol Jpn. 1978; 32(2): 231-5.
  http://www.ncbi.nlm.nih.gov/entrez/query.fcgi?cmd=Retrieve&db=pubmed&dopt=Abstract&list_uids=669498

- **Infiltration pain and local anesthetic effects of buffered vs plain 1% diphenhydramine.**
  Author(s): Singer AJ, Hollander JE.
  Source: Academic Emergency Medicine : Official Journal of the Society for Academic Emergency Medicine. 1995 October; 2(10): 884-8.
  http://www.ncbi.nlm.nih.gov/entrez/query.fcgi?cmd=Retrieve&db=pubmed&dopt=Abstract&list_uids=8542488

- **Inhibition of the gastrointestinal absorption of p-aminosalicylate (PAS) in rats and humans by diphenhydramine.**
  Author(s): Lavigne JG, Marchand C.
  Source: Clinical Pharmacology and Therapeutics. 1973 May-June; 14(3): 404-12.
  http://www.ncbi.nlm.nih.gov/entrez/query.fcgi?cmd=Retrieve&db=pubmed&dopt=Abstract&list_uids=4698569

- **Initial and steady-state effects of diphenhydramine and loratadine on sedation, cognition, mood, and psychomotor performance.**
  Author(s): Kay GG, Berman B, Mockoviak SH, Morris CE, Reeves D, Starbuck V, Sukenik E, Harris AG.
  Source: Archives of Internal Medicine. 1997 November 10; 157(20): 2350-6.
  http://www.ncbi.nlm.nih.gov/entrez/query.fcgi?cmd=Retrieve&db=pubmed&dopt=Abstract&list_uids=9361576

- **Interaction of tolbutamide with phenothiazines and diphenhydramine.**
  Author(s): Iyer KS, Menon A, Moideen TK.
  Source: Indian J Physiol Pharmacol. 1972 April; 16(2): 151-4. No Abstract Available.
  http://www.ncbi.nlm.nih.gov/entrez/query.fcgi?cmd=Retrieve&db=pubmed&dopt=Abstract&list_uids=4404433

- **Interference of diphenhydramine with the EMIT II immunoassay for propoxyphene.**
  Author(s): Schneider S, Wennig R.
  Source: Journal of Analytical Toxicology. 1999 November-December; 23(7): 637-8.
  http://www.ncbi.nlm.nih.gov/entrez/query.fcgi?cmd=Retrieve&db=pubmed&dopt=Abstract&list_uids=10595854

- **Isothermal gas chromatographic analysis of diphenhydramine after direct injection onto a fused-silica capillary column.**
  Author(s): Meatherall RC, Guay DR.
  Source: Journal of Chromatography. 1984 May 11; 307(2): 295-304.
  http://www.ncbi.nlm.nih.gov/entrez/query.fcgi?cmd=Retrieve&db=pubmed&dopt=Abstract&list_uids=6736178

- **Labeling of diphenhydramine-containing drug products for over-the-counter human use. Final rule.**
  Author(s): Food and Drug Administration, HHS.
  Source: Federal Register. 2002 December 2; 67(235): 72555-9.
  http://www.ncbi.nlm.nih.gov/entrez/query.fcgi?cmd=Retrieve&db=pubmed&dopt=Abstract&list_uids=12474879

- **Lack of sedative and cognitive effects of diphenhydramine and cyclobenzaprine in elderly volunteers.**
  Author(s): Lines C, Traub M, Raskin S, Mant T, Reines S.
  Source: Journal of Psychopharmacology (Oxford, England). 1997; 11(4): 325-9.
  http://www.ncbi.nlm.nih.gov/entrez/query.fcgi?cmd=Retrieve&db=pubmed&dopt=Abstract&list_uids=9443520

- **Lethal intoxication with diphenhydramine. Report of a case with analytical follow-up.**
  Author(s): Hausmann E, Wewer H, Wellhoner HH, Weller JP.
  Source: Archives of Toxicology. 1983 May; 53(1): 33-9.
  http://www.ncbi.nlm.nih.gov/entrez/query.fcgi?cmd=Retrieve&db=pubmed&dopt=Abstract&list_uids=6882211

- **Letter: Cleft palate and maternal diphenhydramine intake.**
  Author(s): Saxen I.
  Source: Lancet. 1974 March 9; 1(7854): 407-8.
  http://www.ncbi.nlm.nih.gov/entrez/query.fcgi?cmd=Retrieve&db=pubmed&dopt=Abstract&list_uids=4131054

- **Lidocaine versus diphenhydramine for anesthesia in the repair of minor lacerations.**
  Author(s): Ernst AA, Anand P, Nick T, Wassmuth S.
  Source: The Journal of Trauma. 1993 March; 34(3): 354-7.
  http://www.ncbi.nlm.nih.gov/entrez/query.fcgi?cmd=Retrieve&db=pubmed&dopt=Abstract&list_uids=8483174

- **Life-threatening diphenhydramine overdose treated with charcoal hemoperfusion and hemodialysis.**
  Author(s): Mullins ME, Pinnick RV, Terhes JM.
  Source: Annals of Emergency Medicine. 1999 January; 33(1): 104-7.
  http://www.ncbi.nlm.nih.gov/entrez/query.fcgi?cmd=Retrieve&db=pubmed&dopt=Abstract&list_uids=9867896

- **Livedo reticularis and thrombotic purpura related to the use of diphenhydramine associated with pyrithyldione.**
  Author(s): Morell A, Botella R, Silvestre JF, Betlloch I, Alfonso MR, Ruiz MD.
  Source: Dermatology (Basel, Switzerland). 1996; 193(1): 50-1.
  http://www.ncbi.nlm.nih.gov/entrez/query.fcgi?cmd=Retrieve&db=pubmed&dopt=Abstract&list_uids=8864620

- **Local anesthetic efficacy for oral surgery: Comparison of diphenhydramine and prilocaine.**
  Author(s): Uckan S, Guler N, Sumer M, Ungor M.
  Source: Oral Surgery, Oral Medicine, Oral Pathology, Oral Radiology, and Endodontics. 1998 July; 86(1): 26-30.
  http://www.ncbi.nlm.nih.gov/entrez/query.fcgi?cmd=Retrieve&db=pubmed&dopt=Abstract&list_uids=9690241

- **Long-term heavy use of diphenhydramine without anticholinergic delirium.**
  Author(s): Isabelle C, Warner A.
  Source: American Journal of Health-System Pharmacy : Ajhp : Official Journal of the American Society of Health-System Pharmacists. 1999 March 15; 56(6): 555-7.
  http://www.ncbi.nlm.nih.gov/entrez/query.fcgi?cmd=Retrieve&db=pubmed&dopt=Abstract&list_uids=10192692

- **Massive diphenhydramine overdose resulting in death.**
  Author(s): Krenzelok EP, Anderson GM, Mirick M.
  Source: Annals of Emergency Medicine. 1982 April; 11(4): 212-3.
  http://www.ncbi.nlm.nih.gov/entrez/query.fcgi?cmd=Retrieve&db=pubmed&dopt=Abstract&list_uids=7073039

- **Massive diphenhydramine poisoning resulting in a wide-complex tachycardia: successful treatment with sodium bicarbonate.**
  Author(s): Clark RF, Vance MV.
  Source: Annals of Emergency Medicine. 1992 March; 21(3): 318-21.
  http://www.ncbi.nlm.nih.gov/entrez/query.fcgi?cmd=Retrieve&db=pubmed&dopt=Abstract&list_uids=1311158

- **Metabolic disposition of diphenhydramine.**
  Author(s): Glazko AJ, Dill WA, Young RM, Smith TC, Ogilvie RI.
  Source: Clinical Pharmacology and Therapeutics. 1974 December; 16(6): 1066-76.
  http://www.ncbi.nlm.nih.gov/entrez/query.fcgi?cmd=Retrieve&db=pubmed&dopt=Abstract&list_uids=4447663

- **Methamphetamine and diphenhydramine effects on the rate of cognitive processing.**
  Author(s): Mohs RC, Tinklenberg JR, Roth WT, Kopell BS.
  Source: Psychopharmacology. 1978 September 15; 59(1): 13-9.
  http://www.ncbi.nlm.nih.gov/entrez/query.fcgi?cmd=Retrieve&db=pubmed&dopt=A
  bstract&list_uids=100808

- **Methaqualone-diphenhydramine interaction study in humans.**
  Author(s): Hindmarsh KW, Wallace SM, Schneider CB, Korchinski ED.
  Source: Journal of Pharmaceutical Sciences. 1983 February; 72(2): 176-80.
  http://www.ncbi.nlm.nih.gov/entrez/query.fcgi?cmd=Retrieve&db=pubmed&dopt=A
  bstract&list_uids=6834256

- **Misuse of diphenhydramine soft gel capsules (Sleepia): a cautionary tale from Glasgow.**
  Author(s): Roberts K, Gruer L, Gilhooly T.
  Source: Addiction (Abingdon, England). 1999 October; 94(10): 1575-7.
  http://www.ncbi.nlm.nih.gov/entrez/query.fcgi?cmd=Retrieve&db=pubmed&dopt=A
  bstract&list_uids=10790908

- **Monitoring saliva concentrations of methaqualone, codeine, secobarbital, diphenhydramine and diazepam after single oral doses.**
  Author(s): Sharp ME, Wallace SM, Hindmarsh KW, Peel HW.
  Source: Journal of Analytical Toxicology. 1983 January-February; 7(1): 11-4.
  http://www.ncbi.nlm.nih.gov/entrez/query.fcgi?cmd=Retrieve&db=pubmed&dopt=A
  bstract&list_uids=6834790

- **Neuroleptic malignant syndrome associated with diphenhydramine and diprophyllin overdose in a depressed patient.**
  Author(s): Park-Matsumoto YC, Tazawa T.
  Source: Journal of the Neurological Sciences. 1999 January 1; 162(1): 108-9.
  http://www.ncbi.nlm.nih.gov/entrez/query.fcgi?cmd=Retrieve&db=pubmed&dopt=A
  bstract&list_uids=10064181

- **Nonmedical use of butorphanol and diphenhydramine.**
  Author(s): Smith SG, Davis WM.
  Source: Jama : the Journal of the American Medical Association. 1984 August 24-31; 252(8): 1010.
  http://www.ncbi.nlm.nih.gov/entrez/query.fcgi?cmd=Retrieve&db=pubmed&dopt=A
  bstract&list_uids=6748202

- **Nonorganic insomnia in generalized anxiety disorder. 2. Comparative studies on sleep, awakening, daytime vigilance and anxiety under lorazepam plus diphenhydramine (Somnium) versus lorazepam alone, utilizing clinical, polysomnographic and EEG mapping methods.**
  Author(s): Saletu B, Saletu-Zyhlarz G, Anderer P, Brandstatter N, Frey R, Gruber G, Klosch G, Mandl M, Grunberger J, Linzmayer L.
  Source: Neuropsychobiology. 1997; 36(3): 130-52.
  http://www.ncbi.nlm.nih.gov/entrez/query.fcgi?cmd=Retrieve&db=pubmed&dopt=A
  bstract&list_uids=9313245

- **Oral metoclopramide with or without diphenhydramine: potential for prevention of late nausea and vomiting induced by cisplatin.**
  Author(s): Grunberg SM, Ehler E, McDermed JE, Akerley WL.
  Source: Journal of the National Cancer Institute. 1988 August 3; 80(11): 864-8.
  http://www.ncbi.nlm.nih.gov/entrez/query.fcgi?cmd=Retrieve&db=pubmed&dopt=Abstract&list_uids=3392746

- **Paradoxic excitation with diphenhydramine in an adult.**
  Author(s): Cheng KL, Dwyer PN, Amsden GW.
  Source: Pharmacotherapy. 1997 November-December; 17(6): 1311-4.
  http://www.ncbi.nlm.nih.gov/entrez/query.fcgi?cmd=Retrieve&db=pubmed&dopt=Abstract&list_uids=9399617

- **Perinatal mortality due to interaction of diphenhydramine and temazepam.**
  Author(s): Kargas GA, Kargas SA, Bruyere HJ Jr, Gilbert EF, Opitz JM.
  Source: The New England Journal of Medicine. 1985 November 28; 313(22): 1417-8.
  http://www.ncbi.nlm.nih.gov/entrez/query.fcgi?cmd=Retrieve&db=pubmed&dopt=Abstract&list_uids=2865678

- **Pharmacokinetics and pharmacodynamics of diphenhydramine 25 mg in young and elderly volunteers.**
  Author(s): Scavone JM, Greenblatt DJ, Harmatz JS, Engelhardt N, Shader RI.
  Source: Journal of Clinical Pharmacology. 1998 July; 38(7): 603-9.
  http://www.ncbi.nlm.nih.gov/entrez/query.fcgi?cmd=Retrieve&db=pubmed&dopt=Abstract&list_uids=9702844

- **Pharmacokinetics of diphenhydramine and a demethylated metabolite following intravenous and oral administration.**
  Author(s): Blyden GT, Greenblatt DJ, Scavone JM, Shader RI.
  Source: Journal of Clinical Pharmacology. 1986 September-October; 26(7): 529-33.
  http://www.ncbi.nlm.nih.gov/entrez/query.fcgi?cmd=Retrieve&db=pubmed&dopt=Abstract&list_uids=3760245

- **Pharmacokinetics of diphenhydramine in healthy volunteers with a dimenhydrinate 25 mg chewing gum formulation.**
  Author(s): Valoti M, Frosini M, Dragoni S, Fusi F, Sgaragli G.
  Source: Methods Find Exp Clin Pharmacol. 2003 June; 25(5): 377-81.
  http://www.ncbi.nlm.nih.gov/entrez/query.fcgi?cmd=Retrieve&db=pubmed&dopt=Abstract&list_uids=12851661

- **Pharmacokinetics of diphenhydramine in man.**
  Author(s): Albert KS, Hallmark MR, Sakmar E, Weidler DJ, Wagner JG.
  Source: Journal of Pharmacokinetics and Biopharmaceutics. 1975 June; 3(3): 159-70.
  http://www.ncbi.nlm.nih.gov/entrez/query.fcgi?cmd=Retrieve&db=pubmed&dopt=Abstract&list_uids=1159620

- **Phenytoin-induced movement disorder. Unilateral presentation in a child and response to diphenhydramine.**
  Author(s): Moss W, Ojukwu C, Chiriboga CA.
  Source: Clinical Pediatrics. 1994 October; 33(10): 634-8.
  http://www.ncbi.nlm.nih.gov/entrez/query.fcgi?cmd=Retrieve&db=pubmed&dopt=A
  bstract&list_uids=7813146

- **Photoallergic contact dermatitis due to diphenhydramine hydrochloride.**
  Author(s): Yamada S, Tanaka M, Kawahara Y, Inada M, Ohata Y.
  Source: Contact Dermatitis. 1998 May; 38(5): 282.
  http://www.ncbi.nlm.nih.gov/entrez/query.fcgi?cmd=Retrieve&db=pubmed&dopt=A
  bstract&list_uids=9667449

- **Photosensitivity reaction treated with diphenhydramine.**
  Author(s): Rothschild CJ.
  Source: Can Med Assoc J. 1981 November 15; 125(10): 1085, 1087. No Abstract Available.
  http://www.ncbi.nlm.nih.gov/entrez/query.fcgi?cmd=Retrieve&db=pubmed&dopt=A
  bstract&list_uids=7326639

- **Positive diphenhydramine interference in the EMIT-d.a.u. assay.**
  Author(s): Ajel LA.
  Source: Clinical Chemistry. 1985 February; 31(2): 340-1.
  http://www.ncbi.nlm.nih.gov/entrez/query.fcgi?cmd=Retrieve&db=pubmed&dopt=A
  bstract&list_uids=3881202

- **Positive diphenhydramine interference in the EMIT-d.a.u. assay.**
  Author(s): Kelner MJ.
  Source: Clinical Chemistry. 1984 August; 30(8): 1430.
  http://www.ncbi.nlm.nih.gov/entrez/query.fcgi?cmd=Retrieve&db=pubmed&dopt=A
  bstract&list_uids=6378429

- **Positive diphenhydramine interference in the EMIT-st assay for tricyclic antidepressants in serum.**
  Author(s): Sorisky A, Watson DC.
  Source: Clinical Chemistry. 1986 April; 32(4): 715.
  http://www.ncbi.nlm.nih.gov/entrez/query.fcgi?cmd=Retrieve&db=pubmed&dopt=A
  bstract&list_uids=3513997

- **Prednisone-diphenhydramine regimen prior to use of radiographic contrast media.**
  Author(s): Greenberger P, Patterson R.
  Source: The Journal of Allergy and Clinical Immunology. 1979 April; 63(4): 295.
  http://www.ncbi.nlm.nih.gov/entrez/query.fcgi?cmd=Retrieve&db=pubmed&dopt=A
  bstract&list_uids=429707

- **Priapism resulting from fluphenazine hydrochloride treatment reversed by diphenhydramine.**
  Author(s): Fishbain DA.
  Source: Annals of Emergency Medicine. 1985 June; 14(6): 600-2.
  http://www.ncbi.nlm.nih.gov/entrez/query.fcgi?cmd=Retrieve&db=pubmed&dopt=A
  bstract&list_uids=3994089

- **Primary contact sensitization site. A determinant for the localization of a diphenhydramine eruption.**
  Author(s): Shelley WB, Bennett RG.
  Source: Acta Dermato-Venereologica. 1972; 52(5): 376-8.
  http://www.ncbi.nlm.nih.gov/entrez/query.fcgi?cmd=Retrieve&db=pubmed&dopt=Abstract&list_uids=4117085

- **Protection from nausea and vomiting in cisplatin-treated patients: high-dose metoclopramide combined with methylprednisolone versus metoclopramide combined with dexamethasone and diphenhydramine: a study of the Italian Oncology Group for Clinical Research.**
  Author(s): Roila F, Tonato M, Basurto C, Picciafuoco M, Bracarda S, Donati D, Malacarne P, Monici L, Di Costanzo F, Patoia L, et al.
  Source: Journal of Clinical Oncology : Official Journal of the American Society of Clinical Oncology. 1989 November; 7(11): 1693-700.
  http://www.ncbi.nlm.nih.gov/entrez/query.fcgi?cmd=Retrieve&db=pubmed&dopt=Abstract&list_uids=2681556

- **Quantitative determination of diphenhydramine and orphenadrine in human serum by capillary gas chromatography.**
  Author(s): Lutz D, Gielsdorf W, Jaeger H.
  Source: J Clin Chem Clin Biochem. 1983 October; 21(10): 595-7.
  http://www.ncbi.nlm.nih.gov/entrez/query.fcgi?cmd=Retrieve&db=pubmed&dopt=Abstract&list_uids=6644246

- **Quantitative effects of cetirizine and diphenhydramine on mental performance measured using an automobile driving simulator.**
  Author(s): Gengo FM, Gabos C, Mechtler L.
  Source: Ann Allergy. 1990 June; 64(6): 520-6.
  http://www.ncbi.nlm.nih.gov/entrez/query.fcgi?cmd=Retrieve&db=pubmed&dopt=Abstract&list_uids=1971741

- **Randomized trial of diphenhydramine versus benzyl alcohol with epinephrine as an alternative to lidocaine local anesthesia.**
  Author(s): Bartfield JM, Jandreau SW, Raccio-Robak N.
  Source: Annals of Emergency Medicine. 1998 December; 32(6): 650-4.
  http://www.ncbi.nlm.nih.gov/entrez/query.fcgi?cmd=Retrieve&db=pubmed&dopt=Abstract&list_uids=9832659

- **Reaction to diphenhydramine hydrochloride (Benadryl) used as a local anesthetic.**
  Author(s): Clause DW, Zach GA.
  Source: Gen Dent. 1989 September-October; 37(5): 426-7. No Abstract Available.
  http://www.ncbi.nlm.nih.gov/entrez/query.fcgi?cmd=Retrieve&db=pubmed&dopt=Abstract&list_uids=2637894

- **Recovery after massive overdose of diphenhydramine and methaqualone.**
  Author(s): Wallace MR, Allen E.
  Source: Lancet. 1968 December 7; 2(7580): 1247-8.
  http://www.ncbi.nlm.nih.gov/entrez/query.fcgi?cmd=Retrieve&db=pubmed&dopt=Abstract&list_uids=4177229

- **Relationship between antihistamic activity and plasma level of diphenhydramine.**
  Author(s): Bilzer W, Gundert-Remy U, Weber E.
  Source: European Journal of Clinical Pharmacology. 1974 August 23; 7(5): 393-5.
  http://www.ncbi.nlm.nih.gov/entrez/query.fcgi?cmd=Retrieve&db=pubmed&dopt=Abstract&list_uids=4154042

- **Resolution of the interference from carbamazepine and diphenhydramine during reversed-phase liquid chromatographic determination of haloperidol and reduced haloperidol.**
  Author(s): Vatassery GT, Holden LA, Dysken MW.
  Source: Journal of Analytical Toxicology. 1993 September; 17(5): 304-6.
  http://www.ncbi.nlm.nih.gov/entrez/query.fcgi?cmd=Retrieve&db=pubmed&dopt=Abstract&list_uids=8107466

- **Rhabdomyolysis and acute renal failure following an ethanol and diphenhydramine overdose.**
  Author(s): Haas CE, Magram Y, Mishra A.
  Source: The Annals of Pharmacotherapy. 2003 April; 37(4): 538-42.
  http://www.ncbi.nlm.nih.gov/entrez/query.fcgi?cmd=Retrieve&db=pubmed&dopt=Abstract&list_uids=12659612

- **Rhabdomyolysis: a rare adverse effect of diphenhydramine overdose.**
  Author(s): Emadian SM, Caravati EM, Herr RD.
  Source: The American Journal of Emergency Medicine. 1996 October; 14(6): 574-6.
  http://www.ncbi.nlm.nih.gov/entrez/query.fcgi?cmd=Retrieve&db=pubmed&dopt=Abstract&list_uids=8857809

- **Risk of abuse of diphenhydramine in children and adolescents with chronic illnesses.**
  Author(s): Dinndorf PA, McCabe MA, Frierdich S.
  Source: The Journal of Pediatrics. 1998 August; 133(2): 293-5.
  http://www.ncbi.nlm.nih.gov/entrez/query.fcgi?cmd=Retrieve&db=pubmed&dopt=Abstract&list_uids=9709726

- **Sedation and performance impairment of diphenhydramine and second-generation antihistamines: a meta-analysis.**
  Author(s): Bender BG, Berning S, Dudden R, Milgrom H, Tran ZV.
  Source: The Journal of Allergy and Clinical Immunology. 2003 April; 111(4): 770-6.
  http://www.ncbi.nlm.nih.gov/entrez/query.fcgi?cmd=Retrieve&db=pubmed&dopt=Abstract&list_uids=12704356

- **Sedative effects and plasma concentrations following single doses of triazolam, diphenhydramine, ethanol and placebo.**
  Author(s): Roehrs T, Zwyghuizen-Doorenbos A, Roth T.
  Source: Sleep. 1993 June; 16(4): 301-5.
  http://www.ncbi.nlm.nih.gov/entrez/query.fcgi?cmd=Retrieve&db=pubmed&dopt=Abstract&list_uids=8341890

- **Sedative-hypnotic use of diphenhydramine in a rural, older adult, community-based cohort: effects on cognition.**
  Author(s): Basu R, Dodge H, Stoehr GP, Ganguli M.
  Source: The American Journal of Geriatric Psychiatry : Official Journal of the American Association for Geriatric Psychiatry. 2003 March-April; 11(2): 205-13.
  http://www.ncbi.nlm.nih.gov/entrez/query.fcgi?cmd=Retrieve&db=pubmed&dopt=Abstract&list_uids=12611750

- **Sensitive high-performance liquid chromatographic (HPLC) determination of diphenhydramine in plasma using fluorescence detection.**
  Author(s): Webb CL, Eldon MA.
  Source: Pharmaceutical Research. 1991 November; 8(11): 1448-51.
  http://www.ncbi.nlm.nih.gov/entrez/query.fcgi?cmd=Retrieve&db=pubmed&dopt=Abstract&list_uids=1798685

- **Severe anaphylactoid reaction to radiographic contrast media. Recurrences despites premedication with diphenhydramine and prednisone.**
  Author(s): Madowitz JS, Schweiger MJ.
  Source: Jama : the Journal of the American Medical Association. 1979 June 29; 241(26): 2813-5.
  http://www.ncbi.nlm.nih.gov/entrez/query.fcgi?cmd=Retrieve&db=pubmed&dopt=Abstract&list_uids=448843

- **Severe reaction to diphenhydramine.**
  Author(s): Ramsdell WM.
  Source: Journal of the American Academy of Dermatology. 1989 December; 21(6): 1318-20.
  http://www.ncbi.nlm.nih.gov/entrez/query.fcgi?cmd=Retrieve&db=pubmed&dopt=Abstract&list_uids=2584476

- **Significant interaction between the nonprescription antihistamine diphenhydramine and the CYP2D6 substrate metoprolol in healthy men with high or low CYP2D6 activity.**
  Author(s): Hamelin BA, Bouayad A, Methot J, Jobin J, Desgagnes P, Poirier P, Allaire J, Dumesnil J, Turgeon J.
  Source: Clinical Pharmacology and Therapeutics. 2000 May; 67(5): 466-77.
  http://www.ncbi.nlm.nih.gov/entrez/query.fcgi?cmd=Retrieve&db=pubmed&dopt=Abstract&list_uids=10824625

- **Simultaneous determination of diphenhydramine, methaqualone, diazepam and chlorpromazine in liver by use of enzyme digestion: a comparison of digestion procedures.**
Author(s): Holzbecher M, Ellenberger HA.
Source: Journal of Analytical Toxicology. 1981 March-April; 5(2): 62-4.
http://www.ncbi.nlm.nih.gov/entrez/query.fcgi?cmd=Retrieve&db=pubmed&dopt=Abstract&list_uids=7017273

- **Simultaneous identification and quantitation of diphenhydramine and methaqualone.**
Author(s): Hindmarsh KW, Hamon NW, LeGatt DF.
Source: Clin Toxicol. 1977 September; 11(2): 245-55.
http://www.ncbi.nlm.nih.gov/entrez/query.fcgi?cmd=Retrieve&db=pubmed&dopt=Abstract&list_uids=891115

- **Sleepiness and performance during three-day administration of cetirizine or diphenhydramine.**
Author(s): Schweitzer PK, Muehlbach MJ, Walsh JK.
Source: The Journal of Allergy and Clinical Immunology. 1994 October; 94(4): 716-24.
http://www.ncbi.nlm.nih.gov/entrez/query.fcgi?cmd=Retrieve&db=pubmed&dopt=Abstract&list_uids=7930305

- **Some observations on the EEG. in allergic children: the effects of diphenhydramine. Preliminary report.**
Author(s): Reilly EL, Dees SC, Wilson WP, Musella L.
Source: Southern Medical Journal. 1968 August; 61(8): 874-80.
http://www.ncbi.nlm.nih.gov/entrez/query.fcgi?cmd=Retrieve&db=pubmed&dopt=Abstract&list_uids=5667542

- **Subjective and behavioral effects of diphenhydramine, lorazepam and methocarbamol: evaluation of abuse liability.**
Author(s): Preston KL, Wolf B, Guarino JJ, Griffiths RR.
Source: The Journal of Pharmacology and Experimental Therapeutics. 1992 August; 262(2): 707-20.
http://www.ncbi.nlm.nih.gov/entrez/query.fcgi?cmd=Retrieve&db=pubmed&dopt=Abstract&list_uids=1501118

- **Survival in complicated diphenhydramine overdose.**
Author(s): Rinder CS, D'Amato SL, Rinder HM, Cox PM.
Source: Critical Care Medicine. 1988 November; 16(11): 1161-2.
http://www.ncbi.nlm.nih.gov/entrez/query.fcgi?cmd=Retrieve&db=pubmed&dopt=Abstract&list_uids=3168512

- **Temazepam and diphenhydramine in nursing homes.**
Author(s): Lisi DM.
Source: Dicp. 1989 February; 23(2): 178-80. No Abstract Available.
http://www.ncbi.nlm.nih.gov/entrez/query.fcgi?cmd=Retrieve&db=pubmed&dopt=Abstract&list_uids=2567095

- **The action and interaction of diphenhydramine (Benadryl) hydrochloride at the neuromuscular junction.**
  Author(s): Abdel-Aziz A, Bakry N.
  Source: European Journal of Pharmacology. 1973 May; 22(2): 169-74.
  http://www.ncbi.nlm.nih.gov/entrez/query.fcgi?cmd=Retrieve&db=pubmed&dopt=Abstract&list_uids=4351770

- **The analgesic and hypothermic effects of nefopam, morphine, aspirin, diphenhydramine, and placebo.**
  Author(s): Campos VM, Solis EL.
  Source: Journal of Clinical Pharmacology. 1980 January; 20(1): 42-9.
  http://www.ncbi.nlm.nih.gov/entrez/query.fcgi?cmd=Retrieve&db=pubmed&dopt=Abstract&list_uids=7358867

- **The antiemetic efficacy of secobarbital and chlorpromazine compared to metoclopramide, diphenhydramine, and dexamethasone. A randomized trial.**
  Author(s): Richards PD, Flaum MA, Bateman M, Kardinal CG.
  Source: Cancer. 1986 August 15; 58(4): 959-62.
  http://www.ncbi.nlm.nih.gov/entrez/query.fcgi?cmd=Retrieve&db=pubmed&dopt=Abstract&list_uids=3521843

- **The effect of alcohol intake on the disposition of diphenhydramine in man.**
  Author(s): Calvert RT, Parry R.
  Source: J Clin Hosp Pharm. 1986 August; 11(4): 291-5.
  http://www.ncbi.nlm.nih.gov/entrez/query.fcgi?cmd=Retrieve&db=pubmed&dopt=Abstract&list_uids=3760230

- **The effect of diphenhydramine alone and in combination with ethanol on histamine skin response and mental performance.**
  Author(s): Baugh R, Calvert RT.
  Source: European Journal of Clinical Pharmacology. 1977 November 14; 12(3): 201-4.
  http://www.ncbi.nlm.nih.gov/entrez/query.fcgi?cmd=Retrieve&db=pubmed&dopt=Abstract&list_uids=22437

- **The effectiveness of diphenhydramine HCI in pediatric sleep disorders.**
  Author(s): Russo RM, Gururaj VJ, Allen JE.
  Source: Journal of Clinical Pharmacology. 1976 May-June; 16(5-6): 284-8.
  http://www.ncbi.nlm.nih.gov/entrez/query.fcgi?cmd=Retrieve&db=pubmed&dopt=Abstract&list_uids=770511

- **The effects of acrivastine (BW825C), diphenhydramine and terfenadine in combination with alcohol on human CNS performance.**
  Author(s): Cohen AF, Hamilton MJ, Peck AW.
  Source: European Journal of Clinical Pharmacology. 1987; 32(3): 279-88.
  http://www.ncbi.nlm.nih.gov/entrez/query.fcgi?cmd=Retrieve&db=pubmed&dopt=Abstract&list_uids=2885203

- **The effects of diazepam or diphenhydramine on healthy human subjects.**
  Author(s): Jaattela A, Mannisto P, Paatero H, Tuomisto J.
  Source: Psychopharmacologia. 1971; 21(3): 202-11.
  http://www.ncbi.nlm.nih.gov/entrez/query.fcgi?cmd=Retrieve&db=pubmed&dopt=Abstract&list_uids=5095411

- **The effects of single-dose fexofenadine, diphenhydramine, and placebo on cognitive performance in flight personnel.**
  Author(s): Bower EA, Moore JL, Moss M, Selby KA, Austin M, Meeves S.
  Source: Aviation, Space, and Environmental Medicine. 2003 February; 74(2): 145-52.
  http://www.ncbi.nlm.nih.gov/entrez/query.fcgi?cmd=Retrieve&db=pubmed&dopt=Abstract&list_uids=12602446

- **The effects of sucralfate suspension and diphenhydramine syrup plus kaolin-pectin on radiotherapy-induced mucositis.**
  Author(s): Barker G, Loftus L, Cuddy P, Barker B.
  Source: Oral Surg Oral Med Oral Pathol. 1991 March; 71(3): 288-93.
  http://www.ncbi.nlm.nih.gov/entrez/query.fcgi?cmd=Retrieve&db=pubmed&dopt=Abstract&list_uids=1707149

- **The importance of blood collection site for the determination of basic drugs: a case with fluoxetine and diphenhydramine overdose.**
  Author(s): Roettger JR.
  Source: Journal of Analytical Toxicology. 1990 May-June; 14(3): 191-2.
  http://www.ncbi.nlm.nih.gov/entrez/query.fcgi?cmd=Retrieve&db=pubmed&dopt=Abstract&list_uids=2374411

- **The mechanism of the potentiating effect of antidepressant drugs on the protective influenc oe of diphenhydramine in experimental catatonia. The role of histamine.**
  Author(s): Chopra YM, Dandiya PC.
  Source: Pharmacology. 1974; 12(6): 347-53.
  http://www.ncbi.nlm.nih.gov/entrez/query.fcgi?cmd=Retrieve&db=pubmed&dopt=Abstract&list_uids=4477392

- **The pharmacodynamics of diphenhydramine-induced drowsiness and changes in mental performance.**
  Author(s): Gengo F, Gabos C, Miller JK.
  Source: Clinical Pharmacology and Therapeutics. 1989 January; 45(1): 15-21.
  http://www.ncbi.nlm.nih.gov/entrez/query.fcgi?cmd=Retrieve&db=pubmed&dopt=Abstract&list_uids=2910633

- **The pharmacokinetics of meprobamate following its oral and rectal administration as a series of combinations with diphenhydramine, acetylsalicylic acid, codeine and pentaerythritol tetranitrate.**
  Author(s): Gilbert JD, Aylott RI, Sogtrop HH, Draffan GH.
  Source: Arzneimittel-Forschung. 1984; 34(10): 1323-7.
  http://www.ncbi.nlm.nih.gov/entrez/query.fcgi?cmd=Retrieve&db=pubmed&dopt=Abstract&list_uids=6549136

- **The relative role of brain acetylcholine and histamine in perphenazine catatonia and influence of antidepressants and diphenhydramine alone and in combination.**
  Author(s): Chopra YM, Dandiya PC.
  Source: Neuropharmacology. 1975 August; 14(8): 555-60.
  http://www.ncbi.nlm.nih.gov/entrez/query.fcgi?cmd=Retrieve&db=pubmed&dopt=Abstract&list_uids=1237097

- **The use of flurazepam (dalmane) as a substitute for barbiturates and methaqualone/diphenhydramine (mandrax) in general practice.**
  Author(s): Rooke KC.
  Source: J Int Med Res. 1976; 4(5): 355-9.
  http://www.ncbi.nlm.nih.gov/entrez/query.fcgi?cmd=Retrieve&db=pubmed&dopt=Abstract&list_uids=18375

- **The use of physostigmine in diphenhydramine overdose.**
  Author(s): Padilla RB, Pollack ML.
  Source: The American Journal of Emergency Medicine. 2002 October; 20(6): 569-70.
  http://www.ncbi.nlm.nih.gov/entrez/query.fcgi?cmd=Retrieve&db=pubmed&dopt=Abstract&list_uids=12369036

- **The utilization of diphenhydramine for production of local anesthesia: report of a case.**
  Author(s): Roberts EW, Loveless H.
  Source: Tex Dent J. 1979 August; 97(8): 13-5. No Abstract Available.
  http://www.ncbi.nlm.nih.gov/entrez/query.fcgi?cmd=Retrieve&db=pubmed&dopt=Abstract&list_uids=298103

- **Topical diphenhydramine toxicity in a five year old with varicella.**
  Author(s): Woodward GA, Baldassano RN.
  Source: Pediatric Emergency Care. 1988 March; 4(1): 18-20.
  http://www.ncbi.nlm.nih.gov/entrez/query.fcgi?cmd=Retrieve&db=pubmed&dopt=Abstract&list_uids=3362727

- **Topical diphenhydramine toxicity.**
  Author(s): Bernhardt DT.
  Source: Wis Med J. 1991 August; 90(8): 469-71.
  http://www.ncbi.nlm.nih.gov/entrez/query.fcgi?cmd=Retrieve&db=pubmed&dopt=Abstract&list_uids=1926887

- **Topically induced diphenhydramine toxicity.**
  Author(s): Reilly JF Jr, Weisse ME.
  Source: The Journal of Emergency Medicine. 1990 January-February; 8(1): 59-61.
  http://www.ncbi.nlm.nih.gov/entrez/query.fcgi?cmd=Retrieve&db=pubmed&dopt=Abstract&list_uids=2351800

- **Toxic encephalopathy caused by topically applied diphenhydramine.**
  Author(s): Filloux F.
  Source: The Journal of Pediatrics. 1986 June; 108(6): 1018-20.
  http://www.ncbi.nlm.nih.gov/entrez/query.fcgi?cmd=Retrieve&db=pubmed&dopt=Abstract&list_uids=3712143

- **Toxic psychosis due to diphenhydramine hydrochloride.**
  Author(s): Nigro SA.
  Source: Jama : the Journal of the American Medical Association. 1968 January 22; 203(4): 301-2.
  http://www.ncbi.nlm.nih.gov/entrez/query.fcgi?cmd=Retrieve&db=pubmed&dopt=Abstract&list_uids=5694107

- **Toxicity from topical administration of diphenhydramine in children.**
  Author(s): Huston RL, Cypcar D, Cheng GS, Foulds DM.
  Source: Clinical Pediatrics. 1990 September; 29(9): 542-5.
  http://www.ncbi.nlm.nih.gov/entrez/query.fcgi?cmd=Retrieve&db=pubmed&dopt=Abstract&list_uids=2242650

- **Transepithelial transport of diphenhydramine across monolayers of the human intestinal epithelial cell line Caco-2.**
  Author(s): Mizuuchi H, Katsura T, Hashimoto Y, Inui K.
  Source: Pharmaceutical Research. 2000 May; 17(5): 539-45.
  http://www.ncbi.nlm.nih.gov/entrez/query.fcgi?cmd=Retrieve&db=pubmed&dopt=Abstract&list_uids=10888305

- **Transport characteristics of diphenhydramine in human intestinal epithelial Caco-2 cells: contribution of pH-dependent transport system.**
  Author(s): Mizuuchi H, Katsura T, Saito H, Hashimoto Y, Inui KI.
  Source: The Journal of Pharmacology and Experimental Therapeutics. 1999 July; 290(1): 388-92.
  http://www.ncbi.nlm.nih.gov/entrez/query.fcgi?cmd=Retrieve&db=pubmed&dopt=Abstract&list_uids=10381804

- **Treating diphenhydramine overdose.**
  Author(s): Nash W.
  Source: Nursing. 1994 June; 24(6): 33.
  http://www.ncbi.nlm.nih.gov/entrez/query.fcgi?cmd=Retrieve&db=pubmed&dopt=Abstract&list_uids=8008276

- **Treatment of a delayed reaction to droperidol with diphenhydramine.**
  Author(s): Schreibman DL.
  Source: Anesthesia and Analgesia. 1990 July; 71(1): 105.
  http://www.ncbi.nlm.nih.gov/entrez/query.fcgi?cmd=Retrieve&db=pubmed&dopt=Abstract&list_uids=2363524

- **Treatment of diphenhydramine intoxication with haemoperfusion.**
  Author(s): Viertel A, Sachunsky I, Wolf G, Blaser C.
  Source: Nephrology, Dialysis, Transplantation : Official Publication of the European Dialysis and Transplant Association - European Renal Association. 1994; 9(9): 1336-8.
  http://www.ncbi.nlm.nih.gov/entrez/query.fcgi?cmd=Retrieve&db=pubmed&dopt=Abstract&list_uids=7816303

- **Treatment of haloperidol abuse with diphenhydramine.**
  Author(s): Doenecke AL, Heuermann RC.
  Source: The American Journal of Psychiatry. 1980 April; 137(4): 487-8.
  http://www.ncbi.nlm.nih.gov/entrez/query.fcgi?cmd=Retrieve&db=pubmed&dopt=Abstract&list_uids=7361941

- **Treatment of ingestion of diphenhydramine.**
  Author(s): Borkenstein M, Haidvogl M.
  Source: The Journal of Pediatrics. 1978 January; 92(1): 167-8.
  http://www.ncbi.nlm.nih.gov/entrez/query.fcgi?cmd=Retrieve&db=pubmed&dopt=Abstract&list_uids=619066

- **Treatment of neuroleptic malignant syndrome with diphenhydramine.**
  Author(s): Leikin JB, Baron S, Engle J, Zell M, Hryhorczuk DO.
  Source: Vet Hum Toxicol. 1988 February; 30(1): 58-9.
  http://www.ncbi.nlm.nih.gov/entrez/query.fcgi?cmd=Retrieve&db=pubmed&dopt=Abstract&list_uids=3354188

- **Triazolam and diphenhydramine effects on seizure duration in depressed patients receiving ECT.**
  Author(s): Guthrie SK, Sung JC, Goodson J, Grunhaus L, Tandon R.
  Source: Convuls Ther. 1996 December; 12(4): 261-5. No Abstract Available.
  http://www.ncbi.nlm.nih.gov/entrez/query.fcgi?cmd=Retrieve&db=pubmed&dopt=Abstract&list_uids=9034702

- **Two siblings poisoned with diphenhydramine: a case of factitious disorder by proxy.**
  Author(s): Arnold SM, Arnholz D, Garyfallou GT, Heard K.
  Source: Annals of Emergency Medicine. 1998 August; 32(2): 256-9.
  http://www.ncbi.nlm.nih.gov/entrez/query.fcgi?cmd=Retrieve&db=pubmed&dopt=Abstract&list_uids=9701313

- **Unreported adverse drug reactions determined by screening physician orders for diphenhydramine.**
  Author(s): Fraterrigo CC, Estep JM, Palmer MA.
  Source: Hosp Pharm. 1981 August; 16(8): 421-3, 426.
  http://www.ncbi.nlm.nih.gov/entrez/query.fcgi?cmd=Retrieve&db=pubmed&dopt=Abstract&list_uids=10252375

- **Unusual treatment response of a severe dystonia to diphenhydramine.**
  Author(s): Bailie GR, Nelson MV, Krenzelok EP, Lesar T.
  Source: Annals of Emergency Medicine. 1987 June; 16(6): 705-8.
  http://www.ncbi.nlm.nih.gov/entrez/query.fcgi?cmd=Retrieve&db=pubmed&dopt=Abstract&list_uids=3578980

- **Use of diphenhydramine for local anesthesia in "caine"-sensitive patients.**
  Author(s): Pollack CV Jr, Swindle GM.
  Source: The Journal of Emergency Medicine. 1989 November-December; 7(6): 611-4.
  http://www.ncbi.nlm.nih.gov/entrez/query.fcgi?cmd=Retrieve&db=pubmed&dopt=Abstract&list_uids=2625521

- **Using intravenous diphenhydramine to minimize back pain associated with photodynamic therapy with verteporfin.**
  Author(s): Tornambe PE.
  Source: Archives of Ophthalmology. 2002 June; 120(6): 872.
  http://www.ncbi.nlm.nih.gov/entrez/query.fcgi?cmd=Retrieve&db=pubmed&dopt=Abstract&list_uids=12049608

- **Validation of diphenhydramine as a dermal local anesthetic.**
  Author(s): Green SM, Rothrock SG, Gorchynski J.
  Source: Annals of Emergency Medicine. 1994 June; 23(6): 1284-9.
  http://www.ncbi.nlm.nih.gov/entrez/query.fcgi?cmd=Retrieve&db=pubmed&dopt=Abstract&list_uids=8198302

- **Variability of diphenhydramine N-glucuronidation in healthy subjects.**
  Author(s): Fischer D, Breyer-Pfaff U.
  Source: Eur J Drug Metab Pharmacokinet. 1997 April-June; 22(2): 151-4.
  http://www.ncbi.nlm.nih.gov/entrez/query.fcgi?cmd=Retrieve&db=pubmed&dopt=Abstract&list_uids=9248784

- **Visual hallucinations induced by the combination of prolintane and diphenhydramine.**
  Author(s): Paya B, Guisado JA, Vaz FJ, Crespo-Facorro B.
  Source: Pharmacopsychiatry. 2002 January; 35(1): 24-5.
  http://www.ncbi.nlm.nih.gov/entrez/query.fcgi?cmd=Retrieve&db=pubmed&dopt=Abstract&list_uids=11819155

- **What is the role of diphenhydramine in local anesthesia?**
  Author(s): Green SM.
  Source: Academic Emergency Medicine : Official Journal of the Society for Academic Emergency Medicine. 1996 March; 3(3): 198-200. Review.
  http://www.ncbi.nlm.nih.gov/entrez/query.fcgi?cmd=Retrieve&db=pubmed&dopt=Abstract&list_uids=8673772

Chapter 2. Nutrition and Diphenhydramine

Overview

In this chapter, we will show you how to find studies dedicated specifically to nutrition and diphenhydramine.

Finding Nutrition Studies on Diphenhydramine

The National Institutes of Health's Office of Dietary Supplements (ODS) offers a searchable bibliographic database called the IBIDS (International Bibliographic Information on Dietary Supplements; National Institutes of Health, Building 31, Room 1B29, 31 Center Drive, MSC 2086, Bethesda, Maryland 20892-2086, Tel: 301-435-2920, Fax: 301-480-1845, E-mail: ods@nih.gov). The IBIDS contains over 460,000 scientific citations and summaries about dietary supplements and nutrition as well as references to published international, scientific literature on dietary supplements such as vitamins, minerals, and botanicals.[7] The IBIDS includes references and citations to both human and animal research studies.

As a service of the ODS, access to the IBIDS database is available free of charge at the following Web address: **http://ods.od.nih.gov/databases/ibids.html**. After entering the search area, you have three choices: (1) IBIDS Consumer Database, (2) Full IBIDS Database, or (3) Peer Reviewed Citations Only.

Now that you have selected a database, click on the "Advanced" tab. An advanced search allows you to retrieve up to 100 fully explained references in a comprehensive format. Type "diphenhydramine" (or synonyms) into the search box, and click "Go." To narrow the search, you can also select the "Title" field.

---

[7] Adapted from **http://ods.od.nih.gov**. IBIDS is produced by the Office of Dietary Supplements (ODS) at the National Institutes of Health to assist the public, healthcare providers, educators, and researchers in locating credible, scientific information on dietary supplements. IBIDS was developed and will be maintained through an interagency partnership with the Food and Nutrition Information Center of the National Agricultural Library, U.S. Department of Agriculture.

The following information is typical of that found when using the "Full IBIDS Database" to search for "diphenhydramine" (or a synonym):

- **alpha-Fluoromethylhistidine but not diphenhydramine prevents motion-induced emesis in the cat.**
  Author(s): Department of Pharmacology, Wright State University, Dayton, OH 45435.
  Source: Lucot, J B Takeda, N Am-J-Otolaryngol. 1992 May-June; 13(3): 176-80 0196-0709

- **Physostigmine, sodium bicarbonate, or hypertonic saline to treat diphenhydramine toxicity.**
  Author(s): Emergency Medicine Department, Regions Hospital, St Paul, Minnesota 55101, USA.
  Source: Holger, Joel S Harris, Carson R Engebretsen, Kristin M Vet-Hum-Toxicol. 2002 February; 44(1): 1-4 0145-6296

Federal Resources on Nutrition

In addition to the IBIDS, the United States Department of Health and Human Services (HHS) and the United States Department of Agriculture (USDA) provide many sources of information on general nutrition and health. Recommended resources include:

- healthfinder®, HHS's gateway to health information, including diet and nutrition: **http://www.healthfinder.gov/scripts/SearchContext.asp?topic=238&page=0**

- The United States Department of Agriculture's Web site dedicated to nutrition information: **www.nutrition.gov**

- The Food and Drug Administration's Web site for federal food safety information: **www.foodsafety.gov**

- The National Action Plan on Overweight and Obesity sponsored by the United States Surgeon General: **http://www.surgeongeneral.gov/topics/obesity/**

- The Center for Food Safety and Applied Nutrition has an Internet site sponsored by the Food and Drug Administration and the Department of Health and Human Services: **http://vm.cfsan.fda.gov/**

- Center for Nutrition Policy and Promotion sponsored by the United States Department of Agriculture: **http://www.usda.gov/cnpp/**

- Food and Nutrition Information Center, National Agricultural Library sponsored by the United States Department of Agriculture: **http://www.nal.usda.gov/fnic/**

- Food and Nutrition Service sponsored by the United States Department of Agriculture: **http://www.fns.usda.gov/fns/**

Additional Web Resources

A number of additional Web sites offer encyclopedic information covering food and nutrition. The following is a representative sample:

- AOL: **http://search.aol.com/cat.adp?id=174&layer=&from=subcats**

- Family Village: **http://www.familyvillage.wisc.edu/med_nutrition.html**

- Google: **http://directory.google.com/Top/Health/Nutrition/**

- Healthnotes: **http://www.healthnotes.com/**

- Open Directory Project: **http://dmoz.org/Health/Nutrition/**

- Yahoo.com: **http://dir.yahoo.com/Health/Nutrition/**

- WebMD®Health: **http://my.webmd.com/nutrition**

- WholeHealthMD.com: **http://www.wholehealthmd.com/reflib/0,1529,00.html**

Chapter 3. Alternative Medicine and Diphenhydramine

Overview

In this chapter, we will begin by introducing you to official information sources on complementary and alternative medicine (CAM) relating to diphenhydramine. At the conclusion of this chapter, we will provide additional sources.

National Center for Complementary and Alternative Medicine

The National Center for Complementary and Alternative Medicine (NCCAM) of the National Institutes of Health (**http://nccam.nih.gov/**) has created a link to the National Library of Medicine's databases to facilitate research for articles that specifically relate to diphenhydramine and complementary medicine. To search the database, go to the following Web site: **http://www.nlm.nih.gov/nccam/camonpubmed.html**. Select "CAM on PubMed." Enter "diphenhydramine" (or synonyms) into the search box. Click "Go." The following references provide information on particular aspects of complementary and alternative medicine that are related to diphenhydramine:

- **"Silent" regurgitation and aspiration during general anesthesia.**
  Author(s): Blitt CD, Gutman HL, Cohen DD, Weisman H, Dillon JB.
  Source: Anesthesia and Analgesia. 1970 September-October; 49(5): 707-13.
  http://www.ncbi.nlm.nih.gov/entrez/query.fcgi?cmd=Retrieve&db=pubmed&dopt=Abstract&list_uids=5534428

- **A pilot study of metoclopramide, dexamethasone, diphenhydramine and acupuncture in women treated with cisplatin.**
  Author(s): Aglietti L, Roila F, Tonato M, Basurto C, Bracarda S, Picciafuoco M, Ballatori E, Del Favero A.
  Source: Cancer Chemotherapy and Pharmacology. 1990; 26(3): 239-40.
  http://www.ncbi.nlm.nih.gov/entrez/query.fcgi?cmd=Retrieve&db=pubmed&dopt=Abstract&list_uids=2357773

- **Acute pharmacological effects of temazepam, diphenhydramine, and valerian in healthy elderly subjects.**
  Author(s): Glass JR, Sproule BA, Herrmann N, Streiner D, Busto UE.
  Source: Journal of Clinical Psychopharmacology. 2003 June; 23(3): 260-8.
  http://www.ncbi.nlm.nih.gov/entrez/query.fcgi?cmd=Retrieve&db=pubmed&dopt=Abstract&list_uids=12826988

- **Comparative studies on the effects of the combination drug lorazepam plus diphenhydramine (Somnium) versus lorazepam on the noopsyche, thymopsyche and psychophysiology in nonorganic insomnia related to generalized anxiety disorder.**
  Author(s): Grunberger J, Saletu B, Linzmayer L, Bock G, Weissgram S, Brandstaatter N, Frey R, Saletu-Zyhlarz G.
  Source: Methods Find Exp Clin Pharmacol. 1997 November; 19(9): 645-54.
  http://www.ncbi.nlm.nih.gov/entrez/query.fcgi?cmd=Retrieve&db=pubmed&dopt=Abstract&list_uids=9500129

- **Effects of caffeine and diphenhydramine on auditory evoked cortical potentials.**
  Author(s): Tharion WJ, Kobrick JL, Lieberman HR, Fine BJ.
  Source: Percept Mot Skills. 1993 June; 76(3 Pt 1): 707-15.
  http://www.ncbi.nlm.nih.gov/entrez/query.fcgi?cmd=Retrieve&db=pubmed&dopt=Abstract&list_uids=8321577

- **Evaluation of inhibitory effect of diphenhydramine on benzodiazepine dependence in rats.**
  Author(s): Nath C, Patnaik GK, Saxena RC, Gupta MB.
  Source: Indian J Physiol Pharmacol. 1997 January; 41(1): 42-6.
  http://www.ncbi.nlm.nih.gov/entrez/query.fcgi?cmd=Retrieve&db=pubmed&dopt=Abstract&list_uids=10225031

- **The effect of chlorpromazine, promethazine, and diphenhydramine on swelling of isolated liver mitochondria.**
  Author(s): SMITH EE, WATANABE C, LOUIE J, JONES WJ, HOYT H, HUNTER EF Jr.
  Source: Biochemical Pharmacology. 1964 April; 13: 643-57.
  http://www.ncbi.nlm.nih.gov/entrez/query.fcgi?cmd=Retrieve&db=pubmed&dopt=Abstract&list_uids=14191871

Additional Web Resources

A number of additional Web sites offer encyclopedic information covering CAM and related topics. The following is a representative sample:

- Alternative Medicine Foundation, Inc.: **http://www.herbmed.org/**

- AOL: **http://search.aol.com/cat.adp?id=169&layer=&from=subcats**

- Chinese Medicine: **http://www.newcenturynutrition.com/**

- drkoop.com®: **http://www.drkoop.com/InteractiveMedicine/IndexC.html**

- Family Village: **http://www.familyvillage.wisc.edu/med_altn.htm**

- Google: **http://directory.google.com/Top/Health/Alternative/**

- Healthnotes: **http://www.healthnotes.com/**

- MedWebPlus:
  http://medwebplus.com/subject/Alternative_and_Complementary_Medicine

- Open Directory Project: **http://dmoz.org/Health/Alternative/**

- HealthGate: **http://www.tnp.com/**

- WebMD®Health: **http://my.webmd.com/drugs_and_herbs**

- WholeHealthMD.com: **http://www.wholehealthmd.com/reflib/0,1529,00.html**

- Yahoo.com: **http://dir.yahoo.com/Health/Alternative_Medicine/**

The following is a specific Web list relating to diphenhydramine; please note that any particular subject below may indicate either a therapeutic use, or a contraindication (potential danger), and does not reflect an official recommendation:

- **General Overview**

  Food Allergy
  Source: Integrative Medicine Communications; www.drkoop.com

  Food Poisoning
  Source: Integrative Medicine Communications; www.drkoop.com

  Hay Fever
  Source: Healthnotes, Inc.; www.healthnotes.com

  Hives
  Source: Healthnotes, Inc.; www.healthnotes.com

  Insomnia
  Source: Integrative Medicine Communications; www.drkoop.com

  Ménière's Disease
  Source: Healthnotes, Inc.; www.healthnotes.com

  Morning Sickness
  Source: Healthnotes, Inc.; www.healthnotes.com

  Sleeplessness
  Source: Integrative Medicine Communications; www.drkoop.com

  Vaginitis
  Source: Healthnotes, Inc.; www.healthnotes.com

  Vertigo
  Source: Healthnotes, Inc.; www.healthnotes.com

- **Herbs and Supplements**

    Cardec DM
    Source: Healthnotes, Inc.; www.healthnotes.com

    Dimenhydrinate
    Source: Healthnotes, Inc.; www.healthnotes.com

    Diphenhydramine
    Source: Healthnotes, Inc.; www.healthnotes.com

    Excedrin PM
    Source: Healthnotes, Inc.; www.healthnotes.com

    Tylenol Allergy Sinus
    Source: Healthnotes, Inc.; www.healthnotes.com

    Tylenol Flu Nighttime Maximum Strength Powder
    Source: Healthnotes, Inc.; www.healthnotes.com

    Tylenol PM
    Source: Healthnotes, Inc.; www.healthnotes.com

General References

A good place to find general background information on CAM is the National Library of Medicine. It has prepared within the MEDLINEplus system an information topic page dedicated to complementary and alternative medicine. To access this page, go to the MEDLINEplus site at **http://www.nlm.nih.gov/medlineplus/alternativemedicine.html**. This Web site provides a general overview of various topics and can lead to a number of general sources.

Chapter 4. Dissertations on Diphenhydramine

Overview

In this chapter, we will give you a bibliography on recent dissertations relating to diphenhydramine. We will also provide you with information on how to use the Internet to stay current on dissertations. **IMPORTANT NOTE:** When following the search strategy described below, you may discover <u>non-medical dissertations</u> that use the generic term "diphenhydramine" (or a synonym) in their titles. To accurately reflect the results that you might find while conducting research on diphenhydramine, <u>we have not necessarily excluded non-medical dissertations</u> in this bibliography.

Dissertations on Diphenhydramine

ProQuest Digital Dissertations, the largest archive of academic dissertations available, is located at the following Web address: **http://wwwlib.umi.com/dissertations**. From this archive, we have compiled the following list covering dissertations devoted to diphenhydramine. You will see that the information provided includes the dissertation's title, its author, and the institution with which the author is associated. The following covers recent dissertations found when using this search procedure:

- **CNS pharmacokinetics of diphenhydramine in sheep** by Au Yeung, Sam, PhD from THE UNIVERSITY OF BRITISH COLUMBIA (CANADA), 2003, 188 pages
  http://wwwlib.umi.com/dissertations/fullcit/NQ85977

- **Maternal-fetal disposition, fetal pharmacodynamics and comparative pharmacokinetics of diphenhydramine in pregnant and nonpregnant sheep** by Yoo, Sun Dong; PhD from THE UNIVERSITY OF BRITISH COLUMBIA (CANADA), 1989
  http://wwwlib.umi.com/dissertations/fullcit/NL55258

Keeping Current

Ask the medical librarian at your library if it has full and unlimited access to the *ProQuest Digital Dissertations* database. From the library, you should be able to do more complete searches via **http://wwwlib.umi.com/dissertations**.

CHAPTER 5. PATENTS ON DIPHENHYDRAMINE

Overview

Patents can be physical innovations (e.g. chemicals, pharmaceuticals, medical equipment) or processes (e.g. treatments or diagnostic procedures). The United States Patent and Trademark Office defines a patent as a grant of a property right to the inventor, issued by the Patent and Trademark Office.[8] Patents, therefore, are intellectual property. For the United States, the term of a new patent is 20 years from the date when the patent application was filed. If the inventor wishes to receive economic benefits, it is likely that the invention will become commercially available within 20 years of the initial filing. It is important to understand, therefore, that an inventor's patent does not indicate that a product or service is or will be commercially available. The patent implies only that the inventor has "the right to exclude others from making, using, offering for sale, or selling" the invention in the United States. While this relates to U.S. patents, similar rules govern foreign patents.

In this chapter, we show you how to locate information on patents and their inventors. If you find a patent that is particularly interesting to you, contact the inventor or the assignee for further information. **IMPORTANT NOTE:** When following the search strategy described below, you may discover non-medical patents that use the generic term "diphenhydramine" (or a synonym) in their titles. To accurately reflect the results that you might find while conducting research on diphenhydramine, we have not necessarily excluded non-medical patents in this bibliography.

Patents on Diphenhydramine

By performing a patent search focusing on diphenhydramine, you can obtain information such as the title of the invention, the names of the inventor(s), the assignee(s) or the company that owns or controls the patent, a short abstract that summarizes the patent, and a few excerpts from the description of the patent. The abstract of a patent tends to be more technical in nature, while the description is often written for the public. Full patent descriptions contain much more information than is presented here (e.g. claims, references, figures, diagrams, etc.). We will tell you how to obtain this information later in the chapter.

---

[8]Adapted from the United States Patent and Trademark Office:
http://www.uspto.gov/web/offices/pac/doc/general/whatis.htm.

The following is an example of the type of information that you can expect to obtain from a patent search on diphenhydramine:

- **Analgesic and anti-inflammatory compositions comprising diphenhydramine and methods of using same**

  Inventor(s): Laska; Eugene M. (Larchmont, NY), Siegel; Carole E. (Mamaroneck, NY), Sunshine; Abraham (New York, NY)

  Assignee(s): Richardson-Vicks Inc. (Wilton, CT)

  Patent Number: 4,522,826

  Date filed: February 8, 1984

  Abstract: Novel pharmaceutical compositions of matter are provided comprising analgesic/non-steroidal anti-inflammatory drugs and **diphenhydramine** and methods of using said compositions to elicit an enhanced analgesic and/or anti-inflammatory response in mammalian organisms in need of such treatment.

  Excerpt(s): The present invention relates generally to novel pharmaceutical compositions of matter comprising **diphenhydramine** and one or more non-steroidal anti-inflammatory drugs (NSAID) having analgesic and anti-inflammatory properties, and to methods of using said compositions to elicit an enhanced analgesic or anti-inflammatory response in mammalian organisms in need of such treatment. Non-narcotic analgesics, most of which are also known as non-steroidal anti-inflammatory drugs (NSAID), are widely administered orally in the treatment of mild to severe pain. Within this class, the compounds vary widely in their chemical structure and in their biological profiles as analgesics, anti-inflammatory agents and antipyretic agents. Aspirin, acetaminophen and phenacetin have long been among the most commonly used members of this group; more recently, however, a large number of alternative non-narcotic agents offering a variety of advantages over the earlier drugs have been developed. Tolerance or addiction to these drugs is not generally a problem with their continuous use in the treatment of pain or in the treatment of acute or chronic inflammatory states (notably, rheumatoid arthritis and osteoarthritis); nevertheless, these drugs generally have a higher potential for adverse side-effects effects at the upper limits of their effective dose ranges. Moreover, above each drug's upper limit or ceiling, administration of additional drug does not usually increase the analgesic or anti-inflammatory effect. Among the newer compounds in the non-narcotic analgesic/nonsteroidal anti-inflammatory group are compounds such as diflunisal (Dolobid.RTM.), zomepirac sodium (Zomax.RTM.), ibuprofen (Motrin.RTM.), naproxen (Naprosyn.RTM.), fenoprofen (Nalfon.RTM.), piroxicam (Feldene.RTM.), flurbiprofen, mefenamic acid (Ponstel.RTM.) and sulindac. See also Physicians' Desk Reference, 35th edition, 1981, and The Merck Index, ninth edition, Merck & Co., Rahway, N.J. (1976), for information on specific nonsteroidal anti-inflammatory agents. Also see, generally, Wiseman, "Pharmacological Studies with a New Class of Nonsteroidal Anti-Inflammatory Agents--The Oxicams--With Special Reference to Piroxicam (Feldene.RTM.)", The American Journal of Medicine, Feb. 16, 1982:2-8; Foley et al, The Management of Cancer Pain, Volume II--The Rational Use of Analgesics in the Management of Cancer Pain, Hoffman-LaRoche Inc., 1981; and Cutting's Handbook of Pharmacology, sixth edition, ed. T. Z. Czaky, M.D., Appelton-Century-Crofts, New York, 1979, Chapter 49:538-550, including structural formulas for representative group members. Diphenhydramine[2-(diphenylmethoxy)-N,N-dimethylethylamine] is also a well-known therapeutic agent in long standing use by clinicians as an antihistamine. It is recognized in both the U.S.P. and N.F. as an official antihistamine of the ethanolamine (or aminoalkyl ether) type and is available as the hydrochloride salt in Benadryl.RTM. and various alternative sources in 50 milligram delayed action tablets, 25 and 50 milligram capsules, elixirs (12.5 mg/5 ml) and sterile solution for injection (10 mg/ml). Depending upon the therapeutic indication, **diphenhydramine** is recommended in single or divided doses of between 12.5 to 50 milligrams with a maximum daily dosage not to exceed 300 milligrams. The antihistaminic activity of **diphenhydramine** is directly attributable to its competition with histamine for cell receptor sites on effector cells although **diphenhydramine** also demonstrates, in addition, a number of therapeutic applications attributable to central actions unrelated to histamine antagonism. Antihistaminic indications for **diphenhydramine** include perennial and seasonal allergic rhinitis, vasomotor rhinitis, allergic conjunctivitis, urticaria and as adjunctive therapy for anaphylactic reactions. Central nervous system side effects (non-histaminic actions) which have been capitalized upon include prophylactic and active treatment of motion sickness and, more broadly, as an anti-nauseant and in the treatment of mild forms of Parkinsonism. **Diphenhydramine** demonstrates both stimulant and depressant effects on the central nervous system although stimulation is only occasionally seen in patients given conventional doses with accompanying restlessness, nervousness and inability to sleep. The more predominant sedative action of **diphenhydramine** has been beneficially capitalized upon with the usage of **diphenhydramine** as a somnolent when employed at the maximum 50 milligrams dose in both prescription and over-the-counter forms. In this regard, it is noted that the Food and Drug Administration announced in the November 1983 FDA Drug Bulletin (Vol. 13, No. 3) that **diphenhydramine** (50 mg.) may now be marketed over-the-counter as a nighttime sleep aid.

Web site: http://www.delphion.com/details?pn=US04522826__

- **Antiperspirant compositions, containing certain antihistamines and certain antihistamine enhancers**

Inventor(s): Helman; Michael D. (Edison, NJ), Mackles; Leonard (New York, NY), Rafft; Ronald R. (Towaco, NJ)

Assignee(s): Bristol-Myers Company (New York, NY)

Patent Number: 4,762,704

Date filed: April 28, 1986

Abstract: A topical antiperspirant composition containing an antihistamine selected from the group consisting of antazoline, pyrilamine, tripelennamine, **diphenhydramine**, phenindamine and their corresponding pharmaceutically acceptable salts and an enhancer for said antihistamine selected from the group consisting of sodium sulfate, glutamic acid; octyl palmitate and propylene glycol methyl ether.

Excerpt(s): This invention relates to topical antiperspirant compositions that make use of certain antihistamines. More particularly, it concerns compositions of this character that contain an enhancer for the antiperspirant activity of said antihistamines. It has been suggested in the prior art to use certain antihistamines, alone or in combination with astringent metallic salts, as antiperspirant agents. This is exemplified by two U.S. Patents to Packman et al U.S. Pat. Nos. 4,226,850 and 4,234,566. In addition, in an article by Goodall published in the J. Clin. Pharm., Vol. 10, 1970, p. 235-246, it is suggested that certain anticholenergic or cholenergic blocking agents exhibit varying degrees of antiperspirant activity. Among the drugs that Goodall characterizes an anticholenergic drugs, he includes chlorpheniramine maleate, phenindamine tartrate, **diphenhydramine** HCl and tripelennamine HCl. A somewhat similar disclosure is to be found in "Advances in Modern Toxicology", Vol. 4, Dermatology and Pharmacology, Chapter 1, pages 2-25, edited by Francis N. Marzuli and Howard I. Maibach, published 1977, John Wiley & Sons, New York. One thing that is quite clear from this prior art is that the vehicle from which these drugs are applied is important. The level of antiperspirant activity that these drugs exhibit is very much dependent upon the contents of the vehicle in which they are dispensed.

Web site: http://www.delphion.com/details?pn=US04762704__

- **Aspirin-containing composition including diphenhydramine and an alkalizing agent to reduce gastrointestinal injury potential**

Inventor(s): Lukacsko; Alison B. (Robbinsville, NJ), Piala; Joseph J. (Metuchen, NJ)

Assignee(s): Bristol-Myers Squibb Company (New York, NY)

Patent Number: 5,071,842

Date filed: December 21, 1989

Abstract: A nonsteroidal anti-inflammatory drug composition containing as protectants against gastrointestinal injury, H.sub.1 blockers, H.sub.2 blockers, beta-adrenergic agonists, or combinations thereof, and an alkalizing agent and a process for administering such compositions.

Excerpt(s): This invention relates to nonsteroidal anti-inflammatory compositions containing, as protectants against gastrointential injury caused by said nonsteroidal anti-inflammatory drug (hereinafter sometimes referred to as NSAID), a protectant selected from the group consisting of H.sub.1 blockers, H.sub.2 blockers, beta-adrenergic agonists, and combinations thereof. More particularly, it concerns compositions of this character, that also contain an alkalizing agent, and a process that uses such compositions. The terms H.sub.1 blockers and H.sub.2 blockers are used herein to refer to the histamine H.sub.1 - and H.sub.2 -receptor blockers, respectively. H.sub.1 blockers, H.sub.2 blockers, as well as beta-adrenergic agonists, have been shown to offer some protection against gastrointestinal injury that is sometimes caused by the administration of NSAIDs. These, however, have suffered from some very distinct disadvantages. Among such advantages is the delay in relieving the subjective symptoms of gastric distress that is experienced by individuals who have taken such products. It has now been found that the aforesaid disadvantages may be avoided by also incorporating an alkalizing agent in said NSAID composition containing a gastrointestinal protectant selected from the group consisting of H.sub.1 blockers, H.sub.2 blockers, beta-adrenergic agonists, and combinations thereof. In addition, it has been found that by incorporating said alkalizing agent in the compositons of interest there is often also observed an improvement in the ability of such compositions to protect against gastrointestinal injury that may be caused by said NSAIDs.

Web site: http://www.delphion.com/details?pn=US05071842__

- **Contact dermatitis pharmaceutical preparation with anti-histamine and anti-inflammatory**

  Inventor(s): Santa; James E. (Greeley, CO)

  Assignee(s): Millenium Pharmaceutical Technologies, Inc. (Greeley, CO)

  Patent Number: 5,989,571

  Date filed: July 23, 1997

  Abstract: A pharmaceutical preparation, and treatment method using the same, for contact dermatitis and particularly for canine contact dermatitis. The preparation has as active ingredients an anti-histamine and an anti-inflammatory. The anti-histamine is preferably **diphenhydramine.** The anti-inflammatory is preferably triamcinolone. The preparation is a liquid mixture and is sprayed or otherwise applied onto an affected area.

  Excerpt(s): The invention relates to pharmaceutical preparations useful for treating contact dermatitis having both an anti-histamine and an anti-inflammatory and methods of using said compounds. In one embodiment, the preparation is a composition of **diphenhydramine** and triamcinolone for treating canine contact dermatitis. Human beings and most animals may suffer from a variety of skin irritations and inflammations generally known as dermatitis. Dogs in particular are prone to contact dermatitis caused by flea or other insect bites, allergies, external stimulation such as from prickly plants, and for other reasons. The condition has been notoriously difficult to treat. Veterinarians occasionally resort to injections of various medicines in an attempt to alleviate the symptoms and cure the dermatitis. A number of topical compounds have been used for the treatment of skin conditions for many years. Such compounds have had only limited success in the treatment of canine contact dermatitis. Moreover, such compounds may be messy and/or noxious either to a dog or to a person applying the medicine.

  Web site: http://www.delphion.com/details?pn=US05989571__

- **Coordination complexes of platinum with amides**

  Inventor(s): Roat; Rosette M. (Chestertown, MD), Yolles; Seymour (Newark, DE)

  Assignee(s): University of Delaware (Newark, DE)

  Patent Number: 4,855,498

  Date filed: February 22, 1988

  Abstract: Disclosed are platinum (IV) chelates derived from substituted amides. The chelates result from the reaction under mild conditions of potassium chloroplatinate (II) and the appropriate amide. The chelate transdichloro-cis-bis(dimethylacetamide-C,O) was prepared, fully characterized and exemplified in preparation of the antihistamine **diphenhydramine** hydrochloride.

  Excerpt(s): The invention relates to new platinum(IV) coordination complexes with alkyl amides and preparation of them from potassium tetrachloroplatinate(II) and dialkylacetamides by way of oxidative addition under mild reaction conditions. The product of the reaction starting with dimethylacetamide as an amide ligand was used in a new route for the preparation of a complicated aromatic N-substituted acetamide, an important intermediate in the preparation of antihistamines (diphenhydramine hydrochloride). The importance of coordination compounds and organometallic compounds has increased substantially in recent years with the proliferation of uses of these compounds as catalysts and therapeutic agents. Many of the chemical processes in which coordination compounds are employed are truly catalytic; that is, they are accelerated by very small quantities of the compound which can be recovered virtually unchanged after completion of the reaction. On the other hand, metal complexes are employed in reactions where they serve as starting materials for compounds that cannot otherwise be readily produced, changed in the process, or are not a constituent of the product, so that the metal can be recovered after completion of the reaction. In metal complexes employed as therapeutic agents, a high degree of specificity exists, but as a result of the high level of interest in this field, those highly skilled can determine the biochemical efficacy of a compound from its composition, structure, and physical properties. To appreciate the means whereby the composition and structure of the complex can be varied within the general framework, a review of the basic structure is useful. Coordinating or complexing Lewis bases (electron pair donors) called ligands react with metals (usually heavy metals) or metal ions. The geometric configuration of the complex depends upon the nature of the ligand, including the total number of atoms and the number of donor atoms on each ligand. The position of a ligand with respect to its attachment to the central atom (i.e., cis or trans) may be varied. This can affect the complex's stability and functionality in chemical and therapeutic applications. Coordination compounds are often categorized in terms of the rate in which they undergo substitution or loss of ligands.

Web site: http://www.delphion.com/details?pn=US04855498__

- **Effect of a combination of a terbutaline, diphenhydramine and ranitidine composition on gastrointestinal injury produced by nonsteroidal anti-inflammatory compositions**

Inventor(s): Lukacsko; Alison B. (Robbinsville, NJ), Piala; Joseph J. (Metuchen, NJ)

Assignee(s): Bristol Myers Squibb Company (New York, NY)

Patent Number: 5,260,333

Date filed: April 9, 1992

Abstract: Pharmaceutical composition and process for administering NSAIDs with a combination of beta-adrenergic agonist and certain H.sub.1 -and H.sub.2 -receptor blockers which protect against injury to the gastrointestinal tract. Said composition being terbutaline, **diphenhydramine** and ranitidine.

Excerpt(s): This invention relates to nonsteroidal anti-inflammatory compositions containing, as protectants against gastrointestinal injury caused by said nonsteroidal anti-inflammatory drugs (hereinafter referred to as NSAID), combinations of a beta-adrenergic agonist and histamine-receptor blockers selected from the group consisting of H.sub.1 -and H.sub.2 -blockers and mixtures thereof. The compositions of this invention are useful in treating conditions and symptoms that are classically treated by the administration of NSAIDS, e.g., headache pain, pain and inflammation associated with arthritis and other systemic diseases, elevated body temperatures. Aspirin and other NSAIDs have long been the most popular drugs for the management of pain, inflammation and fever in individuals. However, one of the drawbacks is the gastrointestinal injury and/or bleeding that sometimes accompanies their administration. This becomes a particular problem where large and sustained doses of NSAIDs must be given to control the symptoms, as for example, in the case of the management of arthritis. It has now been found that NSAID-induced gastrointestinal injury can be significantly reduced when a combination of a betaadrenergic agonist and a histamine-receptor blocker selected from the group consisting of histamine H.sub.1 -, H.sub.2 -receptor blockers and mixtures thereof is administered concurrently with said NSAID.

Web site: http://www.delphion.com/details?pn=US05260333__

- **Granulation process for producing an acetaminophen and diphenhydramine hydrochloride composition and composition produced by same**

  Inventor(s): Eisenhardt; Peter F. (Philadelphia, PA), Hitchner; Robert (Perkasie, PA), Parekh; Kishor B. (Horsham, PA)

  Assignee(s): McNeil-PPC, Inc. (Skillman, NJ)

  Patent Number: 5,635,208

  Date filed: July 20, 1993

  Abstract: A granulation process for preparing a solid dosage form containing acetaminophen and **diphenhydramine** hydrochloride, as active agents is disclosed. In addition, the solid dosage form produced by the process is described.

  Excerpt(s): Products containing the analgesic acetaminophen and the sleep aid **diphenhydramine** hydrochloride have been marketed for a number of years. Such products are marketed in various final solid dosage forms including tablets, caplets and gelcaps. The process used to produce solid dosage forms which are then formed into a final solid dosage form generally comprises a single granulation process wherein acetaminophen and **diphenhydramine** hydrochloride together with certain excipients are dry blended and then granulated by spraying the dry blended material with a suitable binder such as starch while the dry blend is mixed in a granulator such as a Fielder granulator. The granulation so formed is then dried, milled and formed into one of a number of solid dosage forms by conventional processing. As used herein the term "solid dosage form" means the solid core component of a dosage form, which may then be processed into a final solid dosage form. In the case of a caplet, it is the core caplet without any coating. In the case of a gelcap, it is the core caplet without any precoat or gelatin coating. In the case of a tablet, it is the core tablet without any coating. Generally, the solid dosage form is the core component formed from a conventional compressing step of the granulation before it undergoes any further processing. The term "final solid dosage" form means a solid dosage form, which has undergone further processing, such as precoating, coating, gelatin coating, printing or the like. The acetaminophen/diphenhydramine hydrochloride solid dosage forms produced by this process possess inadequate hardness, generally about 7 kp or less. As a result, the solid dosage forms may become damaged during processing and packaging. This creates quality control problems and increases production costs. Another problem with this process is that the solid dosage forms produced possess a relatively high friability of greater than 1.0%. Accordingly, it is an object of the present invention to develop a process which produces a medicament which when made into a solid dosage form has an adequate hardness of greater than 7 kp and preferably of from about 9-12 kp and a friability of less than about 1%.

  Web site: http://www.delphion.com/details?pn=US05635208__

- **Methods for controlling perspiration**

  Inventor(s): Jeffkin; Ruth (259 Richards Ave., Lansdowne, PA 19050), Packman; Elias W. (214 Sycamore Ave., Merion, PA 19066)

  Assignee(s): none reported

  Patent Number: 4,226,850

  Date filed: November 12, 1976

  Abstract: Antiperspirant compositions containing antihistamines, such as **diphenhydramine** hydrochloride, alone or in combination with astringent metallic salts, as the active agent effective for retarding or inhibiting perspiration when topically applied to the human skin. Method for controlling or preventing perspiration in humans.

  Excerpt(s): This invention relates to antiperspirant formulations containing an antihistamine, alone or in combination with at least one astringent metallic salt, as an active ingredient and a method for controlling and preventing perspiration when applied topically to humans. Eccrine sweat glands, which secrete copius liquid sweat, are activated through cholinergic fiber innervation, by acetylcholine, which is liberated at the stimulated nerve endings. Apocrine sweat glands are fewer in number and unlike the general distribution of eccrine glands, localized in areas such as the axillae. While the eccrine gland responds primarily to thermal stimuli, apocrine glands are responsive to muscular activity and emotional stimuli. The apocrines are thought to be responsive to andrenergic circulatory epinephrine only. Traditionally, metal salts having astringent properties have been used to inhibit perspiration, particularly the astringent salts of aluminum, zinc, zirconium or rare earth metals. Such salts often require a number of applications over a period of time to reach a satisfactory level of antiperspirant activity. The salts tend to react with the skin, changing its chemical composition and halides of aluminum, perhaps the most widely used ingredient, possess other disadvantages such as axillary irritation, attributed to their low pH, fabric damage and fabric staining. These salts are thought to react with skin proteins, causing coagulation, swelling, and, thus, blockage of sweat glands in a nonselective manner. Difficulty in overcoming these drawbacks increases with the amount of astringent salt used. Also, as reported in U.S. Pat. No. 3,767,786, they are ineffective on some users.

  Web site: http://www.delphion.com/details?pn=US04226850__

- **Microencapsulation process**

  Inventor(s): Cuff; George W. (Indianapolis, IN), McGinity; James W. (Austin, TX)

  Assignee(s): Board of Regents, The University of Texas System (Austin, TX)

  Patent Number: 4,518,547

  Date filed: September 15, 1983

  Abstract: Nylon coated microcapsules containing hydrophilic solvent-soluble anionic, cationic or quaternary drug salts were prepared by interfacial polycondensation techniques. In a first stage, the drug substance to be encapsulated is dissolved in an aqueous phase. Examples of drugs encapsulated are morphine sulfate, **diphenhydramine** hydrochloride, and methantheline bromide. Next the aqueous drug solution is dispersed in an organic phase. In a second stage complementary polycondensation reactants each in an organic phase are added separately, either sequentially or simultaneously, to the dispersion prepared in the first stage. Microcapsules of nylon form around the hydrophilic solvent soluble core drug substance.

Excerpt(s): The present invention relates to a process for microencapsulation of hydrophilic core materials utilizing interfacial polycondensation techniques. The encapsulation of core substances by interfacial polycondensation has been widely used in the pharmaceutical, agricultural, dye, paint, and carbonless paper industries. Microencapsulation is a process whereby small particles of core materials such as liquids, solids, solutions, or dispersions are thinly coated by a separate material. Microencapsulation is often used to improve certain physical characteristic of formulations such as compressibility and flow. In addition, microencapsulation has been utilized to modify chemical release, to improve chemical stability, and to permit the mixing and storage of reactive or incompatible materials. The principle of the microencapsulation method lies in bringing into contact a first liquid phase containing the core material to be encapsulated and a polycondensation reagent, with another liquid phase which is immiscible with the first phase and contains a second reagent capable of reacting with the first to give a polycondensation product. When the two phases are brought into contact, the two condensation reagents react at the interface of the phases, and by polycondensation, a wall of polymer forms around the drops of liquid core materials. The capsules obtained can then be washed and dried before use.

Web site: http://www.delphion.com/details?pn=US04518547__

- **Minoxidil compositions for external use**

  Inventor(s): Imamura; Koji (Kasukabe, JP), Kimura; Fuminori (Omiya, JP), Okajima; Takako (Gyoda, JP), Suzuki; Kenichi (Urawa, JP)

  Assignee(s): Taisho Pharmaceutical Co., Ltd. (JP)

  Patent Number: 6,265,412

  Date filed: November 20, 2000

  Abstract: There is provided a composition for external use with a reduced skin irritation comprising minoxidil and 0.01 to 2 parts by weight of at least one antihistaminic agent selected from the group consisting of chlorphenylamine maleate, diphenylimidazole, **diphenhydramine** and a salt thereof per 1 part by weight of minoxidil.

  Excerpt(s): The present invention relates to a minoxidil-containing composition for external use which, when applied onto skin, has a reduced skin irritation. Minoxidil (2,4-diamino-6-piperidino-pyrimidine-3-oxide), a therapeutic agent of hypertension, was found to cause hypertrichosis as a side-effect, thereby it has recently been used as an effective component in the compositions for external use for the purpose of therapy of genital baldness or seborrheic baldness. However, it is reported that minoxidil-containing compositions for external use, when used, rarely have side-effects such as skin irritation (Contact Dermatitis 1987:17:44). Generally, glycols (e.g., glycerol) and anti-inflammatory agents (e.g., glycyrrhetic acid) are used for healing the drug-caused skin irritation, but they have an insufficient inhibition effect on the skin irritation when used together with minoxidil. As a result of extensive researches in order to overcome the above problem, the present inventors have found that the skin irritation as a side-effect of the minoxidil-containing composition for external use is surprisingly reduced by combining the minoxidil-containing composition for external use with an antihistaminic agent which has been used as a medicine to relieve itching, thereby the present invention has been accomplished. That is, the present invention is directed to a composition for external use comprising minoxidil and an antihistaminic agent.

Web site: http://www.delphion.com/details?pn=US06265412__

- **Multiple action cold/sinus preparations**

Inventor(s): Denick, Jr.; John (Newton, NJ), Lech; Stanley (Rockaway, NJ), Schobel; Alexander M. (Flemington, NJ)

Assignee(s): Warner-Lambert Company (Morris Plains, NJ)

Patent Number: 5,681,577

Date filed: September 19, 1995

Abstract: A chewable cold/sinus preparation comprising a bitter tasting mixture of a decongestant such as pseudoephedrine and an antihistamine such as **diphenhydramine** and/or chlorpheniramine maleate is made with no bitter, metallic taste or unpleasant mouthfeel by adsorbing the active drug mixture using a wet granulation process onto a silicon dioxide carrier which comprises from about 50 to about 85% of total weight of the adsorbate composition. A truly multi-symptom relief formula is prepared through the optional addition of an antitussive such as dextromethorphan hydrobromide and/or an analgesic such as meclofenamic acid, aspirin or ibuprofen. Additional excipients such as flavors, sweeteners, lubricants and bulk fillers are added for better taste, improved mouthfeel and as an aid to the tabletting process.

Excerpt(s): There have been numerous efforts over the years to make bad tasting things that are otherwise good for you taste good. This is particularly true in the area of pharmaceuticals where many drugs possess bitter, acidic or metallic tastes. This problem of course, is confined to those drugs which are administered orally and whereas bitter tastes are readily perceived in swallowable tablets or capsules, they are very apparent and unpleasant in chewable delivery systems such as chewable tablets. The effective taste masking of unpleasant or bitter tasting drugs is important in many respects, not the least of which, particularly in childrens medications, is insuring the likelihood of better patient compliance. Many drugs, both prescription and over-the-counter that are bitter tasting or that possess an undesirable mouth feel can be made less objectionable if they can be encapsulated and swallowed whole with subsequent breakdown and absorption of the active ingredient either in the stomach or enterically in the small intestine. Many drugs however, especially childrens' medications, are better administered in chewable dosage forms since children generally don't like or have difficulty swallowing whole tablets or capsules. Obviously, if the drugs taste bad, chewing the tablet directly exposes the taste buds and sensitive oral tissues to the unpleasant drugs to a greater extent and for a longer period of time thereby exacerbating the problem than if swallowed whole. There are many known taste masking agents and preparations tailored for specific applications. Sweeteners, flavors, bulking agents and the like have long been used as taste masking agents. See U.S. Pat. No. 5,013,716 to Cherukuri et. al. The general approach is using a composition whose taste is stronger than and thereby overpowers the unpleasant tasting compound. Artificial, high intensity sweeteners have proven particularly useful in this regard.

Web site: http://www.delphion.com/details?pn=US05681577__

- **Non-sedating diphenhydramine metabolites**

  Inventor(s): Aberg; A. K. Gunnar (Sarasota, FL)

  Assignee(s): Bridge Pharma, Inc. (Sarasota, FL)

  Patent Number: 6,372,799

  Date filed: February 8, 2001

  Abstract: Disclosed are N-substituted metabolites of **diphenhydramine,** which have been found to be potent and orally active antihistaminic compounds that are devoid of sedative side effects. Phamaceutically acceptable salts of the compounds, a complex with 8-chlorotheo-phylline, therapeutic use and compositions containing the compounds are also described.

  Excerpt(s): This invention relates to new chemical entities as shown below and to methods of treatment of disease states modulated by allergic, inflammatory, or cholinergic activities in a mammal, using said new chemical entities. R.sub.1 is H and R.sub.2 is H or methyl, and the pharmaceutically acceptable salts thereof. The compounds of this inventions have been found to possess pharmacological properties that render said compounds to be useful in treating allergies, inflammations, various types of ocular diseases (such as for example vernal conjunctivitis and allergic conjunctivitis), different types of smooth muscle hyperreactivity (such as for example bronchial hyperreactivity) and asthma or other diseases that are mediated through histaminic receptors of various types.

  Web site: http://www.delphion.com/details?pn=US06372799__

- **Pharmacological composition for preventing neurotoxic side effects of NMDA antagonists**

  Inventor(s): Olney; John W. (#1 Lorenzo La., Ladue, MO 63124)

  Assignee(s): none reported

  Patent Number: 5,616,580

  Date filed: April 26, 1991

  Abstract: This invention discloses mixtures of NMDA antagonists and anti-cholinergic agents, which can be used to prevent excitotoxic damage in the central nervous system or for anesthetic purposes in human or veterinary medicine. Anti-cholinergic agents such as scopolamine, atropine, benztropine, trihexyphenidyl, biperiden, procyclidine, benactyzine, or **diphenhydramine** can be used in conjunction with, or subsequent to, administration of an NMDA antagonist such as MK-801. The NMDA antagonist exerts a primary protective effect by preventing or reducing excitotoxic damage due to stroke, perinatal asphyxia, and various other types of injury or disease; however, strong NMDA antagonists such as MK-801 can also cause neurotoxic side effects, including vacuole formation, mitochondrial dissolution, and neuronal death in certain types of neurons such as cingulate/retrosplenial cerebrocortical neurons. The anti-cholinergic agent will reduce or eliminate those damaging side effects, without interfering with the primary protective value of the NMDA antagonist. The anti-cholinergic agents described herein can also reduce the toxic side effects associated with illegal use of drugs such as phencyclidine (also known as PCP or angel dust).

  Excerpt(s): This invention is in the fields of pharmacology and neurology. It relates to compounds and methods for protecting the central nervous system against neurotoxic side effects of certain therapeutic drugs and against neurodegenerative disease processes. The surfaces of nerve cells in the central nervous system (the CNS, which includes the brain, spinal cord, and retina) contain various types of receptor molecules. In general, a receptor molecule is a polypeptide which straddles a cell membrane. When a messenger molecule interacts with the exposed extracellular portion of the membrane receptor molecule, it triggers a difference in the electrochemical status of the intracellular portion of the receptor, which in turn provokes some response by the cell. The messenger molecule does not bond to the receptor; instead, it usually disengages from the receptor after a brief period and returns to the extracellular fluid. Most receptor molecules are named according to the messenger molecules which bind to them. An "agonist" is any molecule, including the naturally occurring messenger molecule, which can temporarily bind to and activate a certain type of receptor. An agonist can cause the same effect as the natural messenger molecule, or in some cases it can cause a more intense effect (for example, if it has a tighter affinity for the receptor molecule and remains bound to the receptor for a prolonged period).

Web site: http://www.delphion.com/details?pn=US05616580__

- **Sleep-aid composition containing an analgesic and diphenhydramine dihydrogencitrate, and method of use**

Inventor(s): Marcus; Arnold D. (Livingston, NJ), Sheinaus; Harold (Watchung, NJ)

Assignee(s): Bristol-Myers Company (New York, NY)

Patent Number: 4,401,665

Date filed: April 14, 1981

Abstract: An analgesic and sleep-aid composition containing an analgesic (e.g. aspirin, APAP or combinations thereof) and **diphenhydramine** dihydrogencitrate. Discloses several dosage forms including a two layer tablet in which aspirin is contained in one layer and APAP contained in the other layer; the preferred form being such that the **diphenhydramine** dihydrogencitrate is contained in the APAP layer.

Excerpt(s): It is known in the prior art to formulate so-called "nighttime analgesics" consisting of an aspirin layer and an APAP layer; the latter also containing methapyrilene fumarate. A tablet of this character is described in the "Physicians Desk Reference" 28th Edition, 1974, page 640, column 3 (published by Medical Economics Company, a Litton Division, Oradell, N.J.). In these tablets, the methapyrilene fumarate is believed to function as a sleep-aid; whereas, the aspirin and APAP are thought to play their usual roles. These tablets have proven to be effective in the past for their intended purposes. Recently, however, some negative opinion has developed with respect to the safety of methapyrilene fumarate. This led to a search for a drug which might replace it in these tablets. Efforts were also made to use other **diphenhydramine** salts in formulating the aforesaid tablets. Particularly, the salicylate and fumarate salt were employed. However, it was found that with these salts also, the resulting tablets were unsatisfactory resulting in soft, mottled and generally physically and chemically unstable tablets.

Web site: http://www.delphion.com/details?pn=US04401665__

- **Soporific containing lorazepam**

  Inventor(s): Widauer; Josef O. (Allschwil, CH)

  Assignee(s): Medichemie AG (Ettingen, CH)

  Patent Number: 4,590,191

  Date filed: December 3, 1984

  Abstract: A soporific containing lorazepam for oral or rectal administration, containing lorazepam and **diphenhydramine** or a **diphenhydramine** acid addition salt in the weight ratio of from 1:10 to 1:75.The especially favorable weight ratio of lorazepam to **diphenhydramine** is 1:20 to 1:35.The invention also relates to a process for the production of a soporific containing lorazepam and **diphenhydramine.**

  Excerpt(s): This invention relates to a soporific, or sleep-inducing composition, containing lorazepam, for oral or rectal administration. For many people, especially the ill, fulfilling the vital need for a recuperative sleep is ultimately possible only with medicinal aid. This has been for many decades a spur to the new and further development of still more suitable soporifics. Among these, the benzodiazepine hypnotics are broadly used. Representatives of this group with a long half-life result, after repeated use, in accumulation and morning hangover, while the use of benzodiazepines with a very short half-life leads to sedimentation effects and an increased dependence potential. In this group of hypnotics, lorazepam, with a medium half-life, is an important representative. Lorazepam is the unpatented (generic) name of 7-chlor-5-(2-chlorphenyl)-1,3-dihydro-3-hydroxy-2H-1,4 benzodiazepin-2-on. It is known, however, from many years of use of this substance, that its use as a hypnotic is not without problems, since with the giving of somewhat higher doses there are sometimes relatively strong side effects, such as muscle relaxation, ataxia and sedative after-effects, which may occur in the next few days. These side effects are often seen to be intensified, especially in older patients, even with single doses of 2 to 3 milligrams, so that individual doses of more than 1 mg lorazepam may be problematical as to the risk of side effects. Up to now it has not been possible to strengthen the effect of lorazepam without having to tolerate these side effects. A need therefore exists for a soporific which is effective and, at the same time, well tolerated. According to experience, this goal cannot be well attained by increasing the dose of lorazepam.

  Web site: http://www.delphion.com/details?pn=US04590191__

- **System for transdermal delivery of pain relieving substances**

  Inventor(s): Toppo; Frank (1 Corporate Park, Suite 100, Irvine, CA 92714)

  Assignee(s): Toppo; Frank (Las Vegas, NV)

  Patent Number: 5,318,960

  Date filed: June 3, 1992

  Abstract: Compositions for pain relieving non-steroidal anti-inflammatory drugs and/or medicaments such as ibuprofen, methotrexate, capsaicin, **diphenhydramine,** aspirin, methylnicotinate and other medicaments largely soluble in oil, alcohol, and/or water, are produced for transdermal delivery. The composition is manufactured by admixing an appropriate amount of oil surfactant with an appropriate amount of pharmaceutically approved co-solubilizer alcohol to establish a non aqueous phase. The oil surfactant may be a polyethoxylated oil such as castor oil. The co-solubilizer may be isopropyl alcohol or virtually any other alcohols except for methanol. Thereafter, an appropriate amount of distilled water is slowly added to the homogeneous or non-aqueous phase to further reduce viscosity. The final admixture is a clear, oil-continuous solution having a viscosity no greater than 850 centistokes as measured by the VST Hoppler method at 25 degrees Celsius. The composition produced has the capacity to affect the individual surface skin cells (corneocytes) and allow the passage of medicaments to sub-dermal afflicted areas deep within the skin.

Excerpt(s): The present invention relates to a composition, and method of manufacture thereof, for transdermal delivery of pain relieving substances directly to afflicted areas of the body. Debilitating diseases such as rheumatoid arthritis and osteoarthritis afflict 37 million people in the United States. The Arthritis Foundation estimates that 10% of the population of the world and 25% of the population of the United States suffer from arthritis to some degree. Fourteen million work days are lost each year in the United States by arthritis victims. Arthritis is a disease symptomized by painful joints stemming from inflammation in the joint region. Arthritis attacks young, middle-aged and old people alike. Due to the severity of this disease a number of nonsteroidal anti-inflammatory drugs (NSAIDs) have been developed for the treatment of generalized muscle and joint aches, and for the pain of arthritis, aspirin (acetylsalicylic acid), ibuprofen (2(-isobutylphenyl) propionic acid), methotrexate (N-[4-[(2,4 diamino - 6 - pteridinyl)- methyl] methylamino] benzoyl) - L- glutamic acid), capsaicin (8 methyl - vanillyl - nonenamide) and **diphenhydramine** (2 - (diphenyl - methoxy) - N,N - dimethylethylamine hydrochloride) are only a few of the medicaments that are available in prescription and over the counter formulations for the alleviation of pain.

Web site: http://www.delphion.com/details?pn=US05318960__

- **Topical composition**

Inventor(s): Busciglio; John A. (515 Corner Dr., Brandon, FL 33511)

Assignee(s): none reported

Patent Number: 4,748,022

Date filed: December 9, 1986

Abstract: A composition and method of use for the treatment of pain and inflammation associated with lesions of the skin or mucus membrane, such as herpes simplex, herpes labialis, herpes progenitalis, chickenpox lesions, herpes genitalis, sensitivity of gingival tissue due to procedures for etching teeth with HCl, swollen gums, cheilosis, oral traumatic injuries, aphthous ulcer, by applying to the lesion an effective amount of a topical composition comprising **diphenhydramine** HCl, lidocaine HCl, aloe vera gel, propolis and sufficient base to raise the pH to 8-9.

Excerpt(s): The present invention relates to a composition and method of use for the treatment of mucocutaneous lesions by the topical administration of an effective amount of a composition comprising **diphenhydramine,** lidocaine, aloe, propolis and sufficient base to obtain a pH of 8-9. Various agents have been used to treat oral lesions within the oral cavity. Among the most widely used are gentian violet, methylene blue, hydrogen peroxide and surfactants, such as ceepyrn (Cepacol). However, these agents have met with limited success and their clinical efficacy leaves much to be desired. Antihistamines have been commonly employed in dental practice however, mostly for the allergic reactions involving the oral tissues and structures. Among the most widely used antihistamines are ChlorTrimeton, Benadryl, Pyribenzamine and Phenergan. The use of antihistamines has met with very limited success in controlling edema, facial swelling or trismus, etc. resulting from oral surgical procedures.

Web site: http://www.delphion.com/details?pn=US04748022__

Patent Applications on Diphenhydramine

As of December 2000, U.S. patent applications are open to public viewing.[9] Applications are patent requests which have yet to be granted. (The process to achieve a patent can take several years.) The following patent applications have been filed since December 2000 relating to diphenhydramine:

- **Compositions and methods for treating upper respiratory congestion**

  Inventor(s): Gonzales, Gilbert R.; (New York, NY), Jennings, Thomas P.; (Cleves, OH), Schellenger, Norman D.; (Midloathian, VA)

  Correspondence: Wood, Herron & Evans, Llp; 2700 Carew Tower; 441 Vine Street; Cincinnati; OH; 45202; US

  Patent Application Number: 20040122022

  Date filed: December 20, 2002

  Abstract: A composition of an antitussive, a decongestant, and **diphenhydramine** as an antihistamine to treat upper respiratory and oral pharyngeal congestion and related symptoms in a patient. In addition to providing antihistamine effects, **diphenhydramine** also provides effects as an anti-cholinergic, an analgesic, an antitussive, and an analgesic adjuvant.

  Excerpt(s): The present invention relates to the treatment and relief of various symptoms of upper respiratory and oral pharyngeal congestion, and in particular, to a combination medication for treatment and relief thereof. People around the world frequently suffer from upper respiratory tract and oral pharyngeal congestion. This congestion may be caused by allergies, infections in the respiratory tract and/or oral and pharyngeal cavities, changes in weather conditions, as well as from the overall health and genetic disposition of the person. This congestion is generally diagnosed from partially or fully blocked air passages including airways in the lungs, mouth, nose, and throat. Other symptoms related to the cause typically accompany the congestion. Cough, tickles in the throat, cold symptoms such as fever, flu, sinus infections, and throat or gland pain are some of the more common symptoms found with upper respiratory and oral pharyngeal congestion. Congestion of the upper respiratory tract and oral pharyngeal cavity and related symptoms generally have undesirable effects for the afflicted person. For example, the congestion may affect performance in the workplace, school, and at home up to and including loss of work and loss of school attendance. Further, congestion may reduce the ability to perform routine activities, such as housework, driving, running errands, and may even totally incapacitate the person. Severe and intolerable congestion often requires visits to the hospital and treatment. In addition, viral or bacterial infections of the sinus passage or other airway may be passed to healthy persons through symptoms of the congestion. For example, a cough or sneeze may convey a bacterium or virus to another person. Thus, upper respiratory tract and oral pharyngeal congestion and its symptoms need to be treated.

---

[9] This has been a common practice outside the United States prior to December 2000.

Web site: http://appft1.uspto.gov/netahtml/PTO/search-bool.html

- **Delivery of diphenhydramine through an inhalation route**

    Inventor(s): Rabinowitz, Joshua D.; (Mountain View, CA), Zaffaroni, Alejandro C.; (Atherton, CA)

    Correspondence: Richard R. Eckman; Morrison & Foerster Llp; 755 Page Mill Road; Palo Alto; CA; 94304-1018; US

    Patent Application Number: 20030012737

    Date filed: May 21, 2002

Abstract: The present invention relates to the delivery of antihistamines through an inhalation route. Specifically, it relates to aerosols containing **diphenhydramine** that are used in inhalation therapy. In a composition aspect of the present invention, the aerosol comprises particles comprising at least 5 percent by weight of **diphenhydramine**. In a method aspect of the present invention, **diphenhydramine** is delivered to a mammal through an inhalation route. The method comprises: a) heating a composition, wherein the composition comprises at least 5 percent by weight of **diphenhydramine,** to form a vapor; and, b) allowing the vapor to cool, thereby forming a condensation aerosol comprising particles, which is inhaled by the mammal. In a kit aspect of the present invention, a kit for delivering **diphenhydramine** through an inhalation route to a mammal is provided which comprises: a) a composition comprising at least 5 percent by weight of **diphenhydramine;** and, b) a device that forms a **diphenhydramine** containing aerosol from the composition, for inhalation by the mammal.

    Excerpt(s): This application claims priority to U.S. provisional application Ser. No. 60/294,203 entitled "Thermal Vapor Delivery of Drugs," filed May 24, 2001, Rabinowitz and Zaffaroni, the entire disclosure of which is hereby incorporated by reference. This application further claims priority to U.S. provisional application Ser. No. 60/317,479 entitled "Aerosol Drug Delivery," filed Sep. 5, 2001, Rabinowitz and Zaffaroni, the entire disclosure of which is hereby incorporated by reference. The present invention relates to the delivery of antihistamines through an inhalation route. Specifically, it relates to aerosols containing **diphenhydramine** that are used in inhalation therapy. There are a number of antihistamine containing compositions currently marketed for the treatment of allergy symptoms. The compositions contain at least one active ingredient that provides for observed therapeutic effects. Among the active ingredients in such compositions is **diphenhydramine.**

    Web site: http://appft1.uspto.gov/netahtml/PTO/search-bool.html

- **Medicaments for treatmenting colics**

    Inventor(s): Bennett, Basil; (Gauteng, ZA)

    Correspondence: D. Peter Hochberg CO. L.P.A.; 1940 East 6th Street; Cleveland; OH; 44114; US

    Patent Application Number: 20030133998

    Date filed: November 22, 2002

Abstract: Medicament for treating colics comprising diphenhydramine-HCI, belladonna tincture, a buffer and flavourants as well as absolute alcohol, wherein the alcohol concentrate comprises between 2.8% and 3.2% by volume of the medicament.

Excerpt(s): A This invention relates to medicaments. The invention is concerned with medicaments for use in treating babies and in particular to treating babies suffering from colic. Colic is a very widespread illness suffered by babies usually under three to four months of age. Infantile colic is a syndrome characterised by paroxysmal, excessive, and inconsolable crying without identifiable cause in a healthy infant. It is also called persistent crying in infancy and 3-month colic. The behaviour of colicky infants is a cause of anxiety and worry to their parents. Many medicaments for treating this source of discomfort in babies have been proposed but none, to our knowledge is wholly satisfactory. According to one aspect of the invention there is provided a medicament for treating colic comprising **diphenhydramine** HCl, belladonna tincture, a buffer and flavourants as well as absolute alcohol and has been treated to increase shelf life, wherein the alcohol constituent comprises between 2.8% and 3.2%, and preferably 3.2% by volume of the medicament. Where the alcohol is a dilute form of alcohol e.g. alcohol BP 96.4% the amount of that dilute alcohol may be increased so that the actual alcohol content is as mentioned.

Web site: http://appft1.uspto.gov/netahtml/PTO/search-bool.html

Keeping Current

In order to stay informed about patents and patent applications dealing with diphenhydramine, you can access the U.S. Patent Office archive via the Internet at the following Web address: **http://www.uspto.gov/patft/index.html**. You will see two broad options: (1) Issued Patent, and (2) Published Applications. To see a list of issued patents, perform the following steps: Under "Issued Patents," click "Quick Search." Then, type "diphenhydramine" (or synonyms) into the "Term 1" box. After clicking on the search button, scroll down to see the various patents which have been granted to date on diphenhydramine.

You can also use this procedure to view pending patent applications concerning diphenhydramine. Simply go back to **http://www.uspto.gov/patft/index.html**. Select "Quick Search" under "Published Applications." Then proceed with the steps listed above.

CHAPTER 6. BOOKS ON DIPHENHYDRAMINE

Overview

This chapter provides bibliographic book references relating to diphenhydramine. In addition to online booksellers such as **www.amazon.com** and **www.bn.com**, excellent sources for book titles on diphenhydramine include the Combined Health Information Database and the National Library of Medicine. Your local medical library also may have these titles available for loan.

Book Summaries: Online Booksellers

Commercial Internet-based booksellers, such as Amazon.com and Barnes&Noble.com, offer summaries which have been supplied by each title's publisher. Some summaries also include customer reviews. Your local bookseller may have access to in-house and commercial databases that index all published books (e.g. Books in Print®). **IMPORTANT NOTE:** Online booksellers typically produce search results for medical and non-medical books. When searching for "diphenhydramine" at online booksellers' Web sites, you may discover <u>non-medical books</u> that use the generic term "diphenhydramine" (or a synonym) in their titles. The following is indicative of the results you might find when searching for "diphenhydramine" (sorted alphabetically by title; follow the hyperlink to view more details at Amazon.com):

- **NTP technical report on the toxicology and carcinogenesis studies of Diphenhydramine hydrochloride (CAS no. 147-24-0) in F344/N rats and B6C3F← b1← s mice (feed studies) (SuDoc HE 20.3159/2:355)** by U.S. Dept of Health and Human Services; ISBN: B00010GIJG; http://www.amazon.com/exec/obidos/ASIN/B00010GIJG/icongroupinterna

Chapters on Diphenhydramine

In order to find chapters that specifically relate to diphenhydramine, an excellent source of abstracts is the Combined Health Information Database. You will need to limit your search to book chapters and diphenhydramine using the "Detailed Search" option. Go to the following hyperlink: **http://chid.nih.gov/detail/detail.html**. To find book chapters, use the drop boxes at the bottom of the search page where "You may refine your search by." Select the dates and language you prefer, and the format option "Book Chapter." Type "diphenhydramine" (or synonyms) into the "For these words:" box. The following is a typical result when searching for book chapters on diphenhydramine:

- **Drugs Meant to Block Symptoms Temporarily**

  Source: in Haybach, P.J. Meniere's Disease: What You Need to Know. Portland, OR: Vestibular Disorders Association. 1998. p. 163-170.

  Contact: Available from Vestibular Disorders Association. P.O. Box 4467, Portland, OR 97208-4467. (800) 837-8428. E-mail: veda@vestibular.org. Website: www.vestibular.org. PRICE: $24.95 plus shipping and handling. ISBN: 0963261118.

  Summary: This chapter is from a book that provides information for people who have or suspect they have Meniere's disease and want to know more about its diagnosis and treatment, as well as strategies for coping with its effects. Written in nontechnical language, the chapter discusses the use of drugs meant to block symptoms temporarily. The author groups these drugs into three categories: motion sickness drugs, drugs used for nausea and vomiting, and anti-anxiety anti-vertigo drugs. For each category, the author briefly reviews the drugs included, limitations as to who can use the drugs, possible side effects, and strategies for safe and effective drug use. Drugs covered include meclizine (Antivert), dimenhydrinate (Dramamine), **diphenhydramine** (Benadryl), scopolamine, promethazine (Phenergan), prochlorperazine (Compazine), trimethobenzamide (Tigan), diazepam (Valium), alprazolam (Xanax), lorazepam (Ativan), and clonazepam (Klonopin). 10 references.

CHAPTER 7. PERIODICALS AND NEWS ON DIPHENHYDRAMINE

Overview

In this chapter, we suggest a number of news sources and present various periodicals that cover diphenhydramine.

News Services and Press Releases

One of the simplest ways of tracking press releases on diphenhydramine is to search the news wires. In the following sample of sources, we will briefly describe how to access each service. These services only post recent news intended for public viewing.

PR Newswire

To access the PR Newswire archive, simply go to **http://www.prnewswire.com/**. Select your country. Type "diphenhydramine" (or synonyms) into the search box. You will automatically receive information on relevant news releases posted within the last 30 days. The search results are shown by order of relevance.

Reuters Health

The Reuters' Medical News and Health eLine databases can be very useful in exploring news archives relating to diphenhydramine. While some of the listed articles are free to view, others are available for purchase for a nominal fee. To access this archive, go to **http://www.reutershealth.com/en/index.html** and search by "diphenhydramine" (or synonyms). The following was recently listed in this archive for diphenhydramine:

- **FDA Proposes Warning Statement On Diphenhydramine Toxicity**
  Source: Reuters Medical News
  Date: September 02, 1997

The NIH

Within MEDLINEplus, the NIH has made an agreement with the New York Times Syndicate, the AP News Service, and Reuters to deliver news that can be browsed by the public. Search news releases at **http://www.nlm.nih.gov/medlineplus/alphanews_a.html**. MEDLINEplus allows you to browse across an alphabetical index. Or you can search by date at the following Web page: **http://www.nlm.nih.gov/medlineplus/newsbydate.html**. Often, news items are indexed by MEDLINEplus within its search engine.

Business Wire

Business Wire is similar to PR Newswire. To access this archive, simply go to **http://www.businesswire.com/**. You can scan the news by industry category or company name.

Market Wire

Market Wire is more focused on technology than the other wires. To browse the latest press releases by topic, such as alternative medicine, biotechnology, fitness, healthcare, legal, nutrition, and pharmaceuticals, access Market Wire's Medical/Health channel at **http://www.marketwire.com/mw/release_index?channel=MedicalHealth**. Or simply go to Market Wire's home page at **http://www.marketwire.com/mw/home**, type "diphenhydramine" (or synonyms) into the search box, and click on "Search News." As this service is technology oriented, you may wish to use it when searching for press releases covering diagnostic procedures or tests.

Search Engines

Medical news is also available in the news sections of commercial Internet search engines. See the health news page at Yahoo (**http://dir.yahoo.com/Health/News_and_Media/**), or you can use this Web site's general news search page at **http://news.yahoo.com/**. Type in "diphenhydramine" (or synonyms). If you know the name of a company that is relevant to diphenhydramine, you can go to any stock trading Web site (such as **http://www.etrade.com/**) and search for the company name there. News items across various news sources are reported on indicated hyperlinks. Google offers a similar service at **http://news.google.com/**.

BBC

Covering news from a more European perspective, the British Broadcasting Corporation (BBC) allows the public free access to their news archive located at **http://www.bbc.co.uk/**. Search by "diphenhydramine" (or synonyms).

Academic Periodicals covering Diphenhydramine

Numerous periodicals are currently indexed within the National Library of Medicine's PubMed database that are known to publish articles relating to diphenhydramine. In addition to these sources, you can search for articles covering diphenhydramine that have been published by any of the periodicals listed in previous chapters. To find the latest studies published, go to **http://www.ncbi.nlm.nih.gov/pubmed**, type the name of the periodical into the search box, and click "Go."

If you want complete details about the historical contents of a journal, you can also visit the following Web site: **http://www.ncbi.nlm.nih.gov/entrez/jrbrowser.cgi**. Here, type in the name of the journal or its abbreviation, and you will receive an index of published articles. At **http://locatorplus.gov/**, you can retrieve more indexing information on medical periodicals (e.g. the name of the publisher). Select the button "Search LOCATORplus." Then type in the name of the journal and select the advanced search option "Journal Title Search."

CHAPTER 8. RESEARCHING MEDICATIONS

Overview

While a number of hard copy or CD-ROM resources are available for researching medications, a more flexible method is to use Internet-based databases. Broadly speaking, there are two sources of information on approved medications: public sources and private sources. We will emphasize free-to-use public sources.

U.S. Pharmacopeia

Because of historical investments by various organizations and the emergence of the Internet, it has become rather simple to learn about the medications recommended for diphenhydramine. One such source is the United States Pharmacopeia. In 1820, eleven physicians met in Washington, D.C. to establish the first compendium of standard drugs for the United States. They called this compendium the U.S. Pharmacopeia (USP). Today, the USP is a non-profit organization consisting of 800 volunteer scientists, eleven elected officials, and 400 representatives of state associations and colleges of medicine and pharmacy. The USP is located in Rockville, Maryland, and its home page is located at **http://www.usp.org/**. The USP currently provides standards for over 3,700 medications. The resulting USP DI® Advice for the Patient® can be accessed through the National Library of Medicine of the National Institutes of Health. The database is partially derived from lists of federally approved medications in the Food and Drug Administration's (FDA) Drug Approvals database, located at **http://www.fda.gov/cder/da/da.htm**.

While the FDA database is rather large and difficult to navigate, the Phamacopeia is both user-friendly and free to use. It covers more than 9,000 prescription and over-the-counter medications. To access this database, simply type the following hyperlink into your Web browser: **http://www.nlm.nih.gov/medlineplus/druginformation.html**. To view examples of a given medication (brand names, category, description, preparation, proper use, precautions, side effects, etc.), simply follow the hyperlinks indicated within the United States Pharmacopeia (USP).

Below, we have compiled a list of medications associated with diphenhydramine. If you would like more information on a particular medication, the provided hyperlinks will direct you to ample documentation (e.g. typical dosage, side effects, drug-interaction risks, etc.).

The following drugs have been mentioned in the Pharmacopeia and other sources as being potentially applicable to diphenhydramine:

Antihistamines

- **Systemic - U.S. Brands:** Alavert; Allegra; Aller-Chlor; AllerMax Caplets; Aller-med; Atarax; Banophen; Banophen Caplets; Benadryl; Benadryl Allergy; Bromphen; Calm X; Chlo-Amine; Chlorate; Chlor-Trimeton; Chlor-Trimeton Allergy; Chlor-Trimeton Repetabs; Clarinex; Claritin; Claritin Reditabs; Compoz; Contac 12 Hour Allergy; Cophene-B; Dexchlor; Dimetapp Allergy Liqui-Gels; Dinate; Diphen Cough; Diphenhist; Diphenhist Captabs; Dormarex 2; Dramamine; Dramanate; Genahist; Gen-Allerate; Hydrate; Hyrexin; Hyzine-50; Nasahist B; Nervine Nighttime Sleep-Aid; Nolahist; Nytol QuickCaps; Nytol QuickGels; Optimine; PediaCare Allergy Formula; Periactin; Phenetron; Polaramine; Polaramine Repetabs; Siladryl; Sleep-Eze D; Sleep-Eze D Extra Strength; Sominex; Tavist; Tavist-1; Telachlor; Teldrin; Triptone Caplets; Twilite Caplets; Unisom Nighttime Sleep Aid; Unisom SleepGels Maximum Strength; Vistaril; Zyrtec
http://www.nlm.nih.gov/medlineplus/druginfo/uspdi/202060.html

Antihistamines and Decongestants

- **Systemic - U.S. Brands:** Allerest Maximum Strength; Allerphed; Atrohist Pediatric; Atrohist Pediatric Suspension Dye Free; Benadryl Allergy Decongestant Liquid Medication; Brofed Liquid; Bromadrine TR; Bromfed; Bromfed-PD; Bromfenex; Bromfenex PD; Chlordrine S.R.; Chlorfed A; Chlor-Trimeton 12 Hour Relief; Chlor-Trimeton 4 Hour Relief; Chlor-Trimeton Allergy-D 12 Hour; Claritin-D 12 Hour; Claritin-D 24 Hour; Colfed-A; Comhist; CP Oral; Dallergy Jr; Deconamine; Deconamine SR; Deconomed SR; Dexaphen SA; Disobrom; Disophrol Chronotabs; Drixomed; Drixoral Cold and Allergy; Ed A-Hist; Hayfebrol; Histatab Plus; Iofed; Iofed PD; Kronofed-A Jr. Kronocaps; Kronofed-A Kronocaps; Lodrane LD; Lodrane Liquid; Mooredec; Nalex-A; ND Clear T.D.; Novafed A; PediaCare Cold Formula; Poly Hist Forte; Prometh VC Plain; Promethazine VC; Pseudo-Chlor; Rescon; Rescon JR; Rescon-ED; Respahist; Rhinosyn; Rhinosyn-PD; Rinade B.I.D.; Rondamine; Rondec; Rondec Chewable; Rondec Drops; Rondec-TR; R-Tannamine; R-Tannamine Pediatric; R-Tannate; Semprex-D; Silafed; Tanafed; Trinalin Repetabs; Triotann; Triotann Pediatric; Triotann-S Pediatric; Tri-Tannate; ULTRAbrom; ULTRAbrom PD
http://www.nlm.nih.gov/medlineplus/druginfo/uspdi/202061.html

Antihistamines, Decongestants, and Analgesics

- **Systemic - U.S. Brands:** Actifed Cold & Sinus Caplets; Alka-Seltzer Plus Cold Medicine Liqui-Gels; Benadryl Allergy/Sinus Headache Caplets; Children's Tylenol Cold Multi-Symptom; Comtrex Allergy-Sinus; Comtrex Allergy-Sinus Caplets; Contac Allergy/Sinus Night Caplets; Dimetapp Cold & Fever Suspension; Dristan Cold Multi-Symptom Formula; Drixoral Allergy-Sinus; Drixoral Cold and Flu; Kolephrin Caplets; ND-Gesic; Scot-Tussin Original 5-Action Cold Formula; Sinarest; Sine-Off Sinus Medicine Caplets; Singlet for Adults; TheraFlu/Flu and Cold Medicine; TheraFlu/Flu and Cold Medicine for Sore Throat; Tylenol Allergy Sinus Medication Maximum Strength Caplets; Tylenol Allergy Sinus Medication Maximum Strength Gelcaps; Tylenol Allergy Sinus Medication Maximum Strength Geltabs; Tylenol Allergy Sinus Night Time Medicine Maximum Strength Caplets; Tylenol Flu NightTime Hot Medication

Maximum Strength; Tylenol Flu NightTime Medication Maximum Strength
Gelcaps
http://www.nlm.nih.gov/medlineplus/druginfo/uspdi/202062.html

Cough/Cold Combinations

- **Systemic - U.S. Brands:** Alka-Seltzer Plus Cold and Cough; Alka-Seltzer Plus
  Cold and Cough Medicine Liqui-Gels; Alka-Seltzer Plus Night-Time Cold Liqui-
  Gels; Ami-Tex LA; Anatuss LA; Benylin Expectorant; Bromfed-DM; Broncholate;
  Carbinoxamine Compound-Drops; Cardec DM; Children's Tylenol Cold Plus
  Cough Multi Symptom; Co-Apap; Comtrex Daytime Maximum Strength Cold
  and Flu Relief; Comtrex Daytime Maximum Strength Cold, Cough, and Flu
  Relief; Comtrex Multi-Symptom Maximum Strength Non-Drowsy Caplets;
  Comtrex Nighttime Maximum Strength Cold and Flu Relief; Congestac Caplets;
  Contac Cold/Flu Day Caplets; Contac Severe Cold and Flu Caplets; Co-Tuss V;
  Deconsal II; Despec; Despec-SR Caplets; Donatussin; Donatussin DC; Duratuss;
  Duratuss HD; ED Tuss HC; ED-TLC; Endagen-HD; Endal Expectorant; Entex LA;
  Father John's Medicine Plus; Genatuss DM; GP-500; Guaifed; Guaifenex PSE 120;
  Guaifenex PSE 60; GuaiMAX-D; Guai-Vent/PSE; Guiatuss A.C.; Guiatuss CF;
  Guiatuss DAC; Guiatuss PE; Histinex HC; Histinex PV; Hycodan; Hycomine
  Compound; Hydropane; Iobid DM; Iodal HD; Iosal II; Iotussin HC; Kolephrin
  GG/DM; Kolephrin/DM Cough and Cold Medication; Kwelcof Liquid; Mapap
  Cold Formula; Marcof Expectorant; Nalex DH; Novahistine DH Liquid; Nucofed
  Expectorant; Nucofed Pediatric Expectorant; Nucotuss Expectorant; Nucotuss
  Pediatric Expectorant; Nytcold Medicine; Nytime Cold Medicine Liquid; Ornex
  Severe Cold No Drowsiness Caplets; PanMist-JR; PediaCare Cough-Cold;
  PediaCare Night Rest Cough-Cold Liquid; Pediacof Cough; Phanatuss;
  Phenameth VC; Phenergan VC with Codeine; Phenergan with Codeine;
  Phenergan with Dextromethorphan; Pneumotussin HC; Poly-Histine; Primatuss
  Cough Mixture 4; Primatuss Cough Mixture 4D; Profen II; Prometh VC with
  Codeine; Promethazine DM; Promethazine VC w/Codeine; Protuss-D; Pseudo-
  Car DM; P-V-Tussin; Quelidrine Cough; Rentamine Pediatric; Rescon-DM;
  Rescon-GG; Respa-1st; Respa-DM; Respaire-120 SR; Respaire-60 SR; Rhinosyn-
  DM; Rhinosyn-DMX Expectorant; Rhinosyn-X; Robafen AC Cough; Robafen
  DAC; Robafen DM; Robitussin A-C; Robitussin Cold and Cough Liqui-Gels;
  Robitussin Cold, Cough and Flu Liqui-Gels; Robitussin Night Relief; Robitussin
  Night-Time Cold Formula; Robitussin Pediatric Cough and Cold; Robitussin
  Severe Congestion Liqui-Gels; Robitussin-DAC; Robitussin-DM; Robitussin-PE;
  Rondamine-DM Drops; Rondec-DM; Rondec-DM Drops; Ru-Tuss DE; Ru-Tuss
  Expectorant; Ryna-C Liquid; Ryna-CX Liquid; Rynatuss; Rynatuss Pediatric; Safe
  Tussin 30; Scot-Tussin DM; Scot-Tussin Senior Clear; Sildec-DM; Silexin Cough;
  Siltussin DM; Sinufed Timecelles; Sinutab Non-Drying No Drowsiness Liquid
  Caps; S-T Forte 2; Stamoist E; Statuss Green; Sudafed Children's Cold and
  Cough; Sudafed Children's Non-Drowsy Cold and Cough; Sudafed Cold and
  Cough Liquid Caps; Sudal 60/500; Syracol CF; TheraFlu Flu, Cold and Cough
  Medicine; TheraFlu Maximum Strength Non-Drowsy Formula Flu, Cold and
  Cough Medicine; TheraFlu Maximum Strength Non-Drowsy Formula Flu, Cold
  and Cough Medicine Caplets; TheraFlu Nighttime Maximum Strength Flu, Cold
  and Cough; Tolu-Sed DM; Touro DM; Touro LA Caplets; Triacin C Cough;
  Triafed w/Codeine; Triaminic AM Non-Drowsy Cough and Decongestant;
  Triaminic Night Time; Triaminic Sore Throat Formula; Tri-Tannate Plus
  Pediatric; Tussafed; Tussafed Drops; Tussar DM; Tussigon; Tussionex

Pennkinetic; Tussi-Organidin DM NR Liquid; Tussi-Organidin DM-S NR Liquid; Tussi-Organidin NR Liquid; Tussi-Organidin-S NR Liquid; Tussirex; Tuss-LA; Tusso-DM; Tylenol Cold and Flu No Drowsiness Powder; Tylenol Cold Medication; Tylenol Cold Medication Caplets; Tylenol Cold Medication, Non-Drowsy Caplets; Tylenol Cold Medication, Non-Drowsy Gelcaps; Tylenol Cold Multi-Symptom; Tylenol Maximum Strength Flu Gelcaps; Tylenol Multi-Symptom Cough; Uni-tussin DM; Vanex-HD; V-Dec-M; Versacaps; Vicks 44 Cough and Cold Relief Non-Drowsy LiquiCaps; Vicks 44D Cough and Head Congestion; Vicks 44E Cough and Chest Congestion; Vicks 44M Cough, Cold and Flu Relief; Vicks Children's Cough Syrup; Vicks Children's NyQuil Cold/Cough Relief; Vicks DayQuil Multi-Symptom Cold/Flu LiquiCaps; Vicks DayQuil Multi-Symptom Cold/Flu Relief; Vicks NyQuil Hot Therapy; Vicks NyQuil Multi-Symptom Cold/Flu LiquiCaps; Vicks NyQuil Multi-Symptom Cold/Flu Relief; Vicks Pediatric 44D Cough and Head Decongestion; Vicks Pediatric 44M Multi-Symptom Cough and Cold; Vicodin Tuss; Zephrex; Zephrex-LA
http://www.nlm.nih.gov/medlineplus/druginfo/uspdi/202165.html

Headache Medicines, Ergot Derivative-Containing

- **Systemic - U.S. Brands:** Cafergot; Cafertine; Cafetrate; D.H.E. 45; Ercaf; Ergo-Caff; Ergomar; Ergostat; Gotamine; Migergot; Wigraine
http://www.nlm.nih.gov/medlineplus/druginfo/uspdi/202216.html

Commercial Databases

In addition to the medications listed in the USP above, a number of commercial sites are available by subscription to physicians and their institutions. Or, you may be able to access these sources from your local medical library.

Mosby's Drug Consult™

Mosby's Drug Consult™ database (also available on CD-ROM and book format) covers 45,000 drug products including generics and international brands. It provides prescribing information, drug interactions, and patient information. Subscription information is available at the following hyperlink: **http://www.mosbysdrugconsult.com/**.

PDR*health*

The PDR*health* database is a free-to-use, drug information search engine that has been written for the public in layman's terms. It contains FDA-approved drug information adapted from the Physicians' Desk Reference (PDR) database. PDR*health* can be searched by brand name, generic name, or indication. It features multiple drug interactions reports. Search PDR*health* at **http://www.pdrhealth.com/drug_info/index.html**.

Other Web Sites

Drugs.com (**www.drugs.com**) reproduces the information in the Pharmacopeia as well as commercial information. You may also want to consider the Web site of the Medical Letter, Inc. (**http://www.medletter.com/**) which allows users to download articles on various drugs and therapeutics for a nominal fee.

If you have any questions about a medical treatment, the FDA may have an office near you. Look for their number in the blue pages of the phone book. You can also contact the FDA through its toll-free number, 1-888-INFO-FDA (1-888-463-6332), or on the World Wide Web at **www.fda.gov**.

APPENDICES

APPENDIX A. PHYSICIAN RESOURCES

Overview

In this chapter, we focus on databases and Internet-based guidelines and information resources created or written for a professional audience.

NIH Guidelines

Commonly referred to as "clinical" or "professional" guidelines, the National Institutes of Health publish physician guidelines for the most common diseases. Publications are available at the following by relevant Institute[10]:

- Office of the Director (OD); guidelines consolidated across agencies available at **http://www.nih.gov/health/consumer/conkey.htm**

- National Institute of General Medical Sciences (NIGMS); fact sheets available at **http://www.nigms.nih.gov/news/facts/**

- National Library of Medicine (NLM); extensive encyclopedia (A.D.A.M., Inc.) with guidelines: **http://www.nlm.nih.gov/medlineplus/healthtopics.html**

- National Cancer Institute (NCI); guidelines available at **http://www.cancer.gov/cancerinfo/list.aspx?viewid=5f35036e-5497-4d86-8c2c-714a9f7c8d25**

- National Eye Institute (NEI); guidelines available at **http://www.nei.nih.gov/order/index.htm**

- National Heart, Lung, and Blood Institute (NHLBI); guidelines available at **http://www.nhlbi.nih.gov/guidelines/index.htm**

- National Human Genome Research Institute (NHGRI); research available at **http://www.genome.gov/page.cfm?pageID=10000375**

- National Institute on Aging (NIA); guidelines available at **http://www.nia.nih.gov/health/**

---

[10] These publications are typically written by one or more of the various NIH Institutes.

- National Institute on Alcohol Abuse and Alcoholism (NIAAA); guidelines available at **http://www.niaaa.nih.gov/publications/publications.htm**

- National Institute of Allergy and Infectious Diseases (NIAID); guidelines available at **http://www.niaid.nih.gov/publications/**

- National Institute of Arthritis and Musculoskeletal and Skin Diseases (NIAMS); fact sheets and guidelines available at **http://www.niams.nih.gov/hi/index.htm**

- National Institute of Child Health and Human Development (NICHD); guidelines available at **http://www.nichd.nih.gov/publications/pubskey.cfm**

- National Institute on Deafness and Other Communication Disorders (NIDCD); fact sheets and guidelines at **http://www.nidcd.nih.gov/health/**

- National Institute of Dental and Craniofacial Research (NIDCR); guidelines available at **http://www.nidr.nih.gov/health/**

- National Institute of Diabetes and Digestive and Kidney Diseases (NIDDK); guidelines available at **http://www.niddk.nih.gov/health/health.htm**

- National Institute on Drug Abuse (NIDA); guidelines available at **http://www.nida.nih.gov/DrugAbuse.html**

- National Institute of Environmental Health Sciences (NIEHS); environmental health information available at **http://www.niehs.nih.gov/external/facts.htm**

- National Institute of Mental Health (NIMH); guidelines available at **http://www.nimh.nih.gov/practitioners/index.cfm**

- National Institute of Neurological Disorders and Stroke (NINDS); neurological disorder information pages available at **http://www.ninds.nih.gov/health_and_medical/disorder_index.htm**

- National Institute of Nursing Research (NINR); publications on selected illnesses at **http://www.nih.gov/ninr/news-info/publications.html**

- National Institute of Biomedical Imaging and Bioengineering; general information at **http://grants.nih.gov/grants/becon/becon_info.htm**

- Center for Information Technology (CIT); referrals to other agencies based on keyword searches available at **http://kb.nih.gov/www_query_main.asp**

- National Center for Complementary and Alternative Medicine (NCCAM); health information available at **http://nccam.nih.gov/health/**

- National Center for Research Resources (NCRR); various information directories available at **http://www.ncrr.nih.gov/publications.asp**

- Office of Rare Diseases; various fact sheets available at **http://rarediseases.info.nih.gov/html/resources/rep_pubs.html**

- Centers for Disease Control and Prevention; various fact sheets on infectious diseases available at **http://www.cdc.gov/publications.htm**

NIH Databases

In addition to the various Institutes of Health that publish professional guidelines, the NIH has designed a number of databases for professionals.[11] Physician-oriented resources provide a wide variety of information related to the biomedical and health sciences, both past and present. The format of these resources varies. Searchable databases, bibliographic citations, full-text articles (when available), archival collections, and images are all available. The following are referenced by the National Library of Medicine:[12]

- **Bioethics:** Access to published literature on the ethical, legal, and public policy issues surrounding healthcare and biomedical research. This information is provided in conjunction with the Kennedy Institute of Ethics located at Georgetown University, Washington, D.C.: **http://www.nlm.nih.gov/databases/databases_bioethics.html**

- **HIV/AIDS Resources:** Describes various links and databases dedicated to HIV/AIDS research: **http://www.nlm.nih.gov/pubs/factsheets/aidsinfs.html**

- **NLM Online Exhibitions:** Describes "Exhibitions in the History of Medicine": **http://www.nlm.nih.gov/exhibition/exhibition.html**. Additional resources for historical scholarship in medicine: **http://www.nlm.nih.gov/hmd/hmd.html**

- **Biotechnology Information:** Access to public databases. The National Center for Biotechnology Information conducts research in computational biology, develops software tools for analyzing genome data, and disseminates biomedical information for the better understanding of molecular processes affecting human health and disease: **http://www.ncbi.nlm.nih.gov/**

- **Population Information:** The National Library of Medicine provides access to worldwide coverage of population, family planning, and related health issues, including family planning technology and programs, fertility, and population law and policy: **http://www.nlm.nih.gov/databases/databases_population.html**

- **Cancer Information:** Access to cancer-oriented databases: **http://www.nlm.nih.gov/databases/databases_cancer.html**

- **Profiles in Science:** Offering the archival collections of prominent twentieth-century biomedical scientists to the public through modern digital technology: **http://www.profiles.nlm.nih.gov/**

- **Chemical Information:** Provides links to various chemical databases and references: **http://sis.nlm.nih.gov/Chem/ChemMain.html**

- **Clinical Alerts:** Reports the release of findings from the NIH-funded clinical trials where such release could significantly affect morbidity and mortality: **http://www.nlm.nih.gov/databases/alerts/clinical_alerts.html**

- **Space Life Sciences:** Provides links and information to space-based research (including NASA): **http://www.nlm.nih.gov/databases/databases_space.html**

- **MEDLINE:** Bibliographic database covering the fields of medicine, nursing, dentistry, veterinary medicine, the healthcare system, and the pre-clinical sciences: **http://www.nlm.nih.gov/databases/databases_medline.html**

---

[11] Remember, for the general public, the National Library of Medicine recommends the databases referenced in MEDLINE*plus* (**http://medlineplus.gov/** or **http://www.nlm.nih.gov/medlineplus/databases.html**).

[12] See **http://www.nlm.nih.gov/databases/databases.html**.

- **Toxicology and Environmental Health Information (TOXNET):** Databases covering toxicology and environmental health: **http://sis.nlm.nih.gov/Tox/ToxMain.html**

- **Visible Human Interface:** Anatomically detailed, three-dimensional representations of normal male and female human bodies: **http://www.nlm.nih.gov/research/visible/visible_human.html**

The NLM Gateway[13]

The NLM (National Library of Medicine) Gateway is a Web-based system that lets users search simultaneously in multiple retrieval systems at the U.S. National Library of Medicine (NLM). It allows users of NLM services to initiate searches from one Web interface, providing one-stop searching for many of NLM's information resources or databases.[14] To use the NLM Gateway, simply go to the search site at **http://gateway.nlm.nih.gov/gw/Cmd**. Type "diphenhydramine" (or synonyms) into the search box and click "Search." The results will be presented in a tabular form, indicating the number of references in each database category.

Results Summary

Category	Items Found
Journal Articles	4849
Books / Periodicals / Audio Visual	5
Consumer Health	997
Meeting Abstracts	10
Other Collections	124
Total	5985

HSTAT[15]

HSTAT is a free, Web-based resource that provides access to full-text documents used in healthcare decision-making.[16] These documents include clinical practice guidelines, quick-reference guides for clinicians, consumer health brochures, evidence reports and technology assessments from the Agency for Healthcare Research and Quality (AHRQ), as well as AHRQ's Put Prevention Into Practice.[17] Simply search by "diphenhydramine" (or synonyms) at the following Web site: **http://text.nlm.nih.gov**.

---

[13] Adapted from NLM: **http://gateway.nlm.nih.gov/gw/Cmd?Overview.x**.

[14] The NLM Gateway is currently being developed by the Lister Hill National Center for Biomedical Communications (LHNCBC) at the National Library of Medicine (NLM) of the National Institutes of Health (NIH).

[15] Adapted from HSTAT: **http://www.nlm.nih.gov/pubs/factsheets/hstat.html**.

[16] The HSTAT URL is **http://hstat.nlm.nih.gov/**.

[17] Other important documents in HSTAT include: the National Institutes of Health (NIH) Consensus Conference Reports and Technology Assessment Reports; the HIV/AIDS Treatment Information Service (ATIS) resource documents; the Substance Abuse and Mental Health Services Administration's Center for Substance Abuse Treatment (SAMHSA/CSAT) Treatment Improvement Protocols (TIP) and Center for Substance Abuse Prevention (SAMHSA/CSAP) Prevention Enhancement Protocols System (PEPS); the Public Health Service (PHS) Preventive Services Task Force's *Guide to Clinical Preventive Services*; the independent, nonfederal Task Force on Community Services' *Guide to Community Preventive Services*; and the Health Technology Advisory Committee (HTAC) of the Minnesota Health Care Commission (MHCC) health technology evaluations.

Coffee Break: Tutorials for Biologists[18]

Coffee Break is a general healthcare site that takes a scientific view of the news and covers recent breakthroughs in biology that may one day assist physicians in developing treatments. Here you will find a collection of short reports on recent biological discoveries. Each report incorporates interactive tutorials that demonstrate how bioinformatics tools are used as a part of the research process. Currently, all Coffee Breaks are written by NCBI staff.[19] Each report is about 400 words and is usually based on a discovery reported in one or more articles from recently published, peer-reviewed literature.[20] This site has new articles every few weeks, so it can be considered an online magazine of sorts. It is intended for general background information. You can access the Coffee Break Web site at the following hyperlink: **http://www.ncbi.nlm.nih.gov/Coffeebreak/**.

Other Commercial Databases

In addition to resources maintained by official agencies, other databases exist that are commercial ventures addressing medical professionals. Here are some examples that may interest you:

- **CliniWeb International:** Index and table of contents to selected clinical information on the Internet; see **http://www.ohsu.edu/cliniweb/**.

- **Medical World Search:** Searches full text from thousands of selected medical sites on the Internet; see **http://www.mwsearch.com/**.

---

[18] Adapted from **http://www.ncbi.nlm.nih.gov/Coffeebreak/Archive/FAQ.html**.

[19] The figure that accompanies each article is frequently supplied by an expert external to NCBI, in which case the source of the figure is cited. The result is an interactive tutorial that tells a biological story.

[20] After a brief introduction that sets the work described into a broader context, the report focuses on how a molecular understanding can provide explanations of observed biology and lead to therapies for diseases. Each vignette is accompanied by a figure and hypertext links that lead to a series of pages that interactively show how NCBI tools and resources are used in the research process.

APPENDIX B. PATIENT RESOURCES

Overview

Official agencies, as well as federally funded institutions supported by national grants, frequently publish a variety of guidelines written with the patient in mind. These are typically called "Fact Sheets" or "Guidelines." They can take the form of a brochure, information kit, pamphlet, or flyer. Often they are only a few pages in length. Since new guidelines on diphenhydramine can appear at any moment and be published by a number of sources, the best approach to finding guidelines is to systematically scan the Internet-based services that post them.

Patient Guideline Sources

The remainder of this chapter directs you to sources which either publish or can help you find additional guidelines on topics related to diphenhydramine. Due to space limitations, these sources are listed in a concise manner. Do not hesitate to consult the following sources by either using the Internet hyperlink provided, or, in cases where the contact information is provided, contacting the publisher or author directly.

The National Institutes of Health

The NIH gateway to patients is located at **http://health.nih.gov/**. From this site, you can search across various sources and institutes, a number of which are summarized below.

Topic Pages: MEDLINEplus

The National Library of Medicine has created a vast and patient-oriented healthcare information portal called MEDLINEplus. Within this Internet-based system are "health topic pages" which list links to available materials relevant to diphenhydramine. To access this system, log on to **http://www.nlm.nih.gov/medlineplus/healthtopics.html**. From there you can either search using the alphabetical index or browse by broad topic areas. Recently, MEDLINEplus listed the following when searched for "diphenhydramine":

Hives
http://www.nlm.nih.gov/medlineplus/hives.html

Nose Disorders
http://www.nlm.nih.gov/medlineplus/nosedisorders.html

Sinusitis
http://www.nlm.nih.gov/medlineplus/sinusitis.html

You may also choose to use the search utility provided by MEDLINEplus at the following Web address: **http://www.nlm.nih.gov/medlineplus/**. Simply type a keyword into the search box and click "Search." This utility is similar to the NIH search utility, with the exception that it only includes materials that are linked within the MEDLINEplus system (mostly patient-oriented information). It also has the disadvantage of generating unstructured results. We recommend, therefore, that you use this method only if you have a very targeted search.

The NIH Search Utility

The NIH search utility allows you to search for documents on over 100 selected Web sites that comprise the NIH-WEB-SPACE. Each of these servers is "crawled" and indexed on an ongoing basis. Your search will produce a list of various documents, all of which will relate in some way to diphenhydramine. The drawbacks of this approach are that the information is not organized by theme and that the references are often a mix of information for professionals and patients. Nevertheless, a large number of the listed Web sites provide useful background information. We can only recommend this route, therefore, for relatively rare or specific disorders, or when using highly targeted searches. To use the NIH search utility, visit the following Web page: **http://search.nih.gov/index.html**.

Additional Web Sources

A number of Web sites are available to the public that often link to government sites. These can also point you in the direction of essential information. The following is a representative sample:

- AOL: **http://search.aol.com/cat.adp?id=168&layer=&from=subcats**

- Family Village: **http://www.familyvillage.wisc.edu/specific.htm**

- Google: **http://directory.google.com/Top/Health/Conditions_and_Diseases/**

- Med Help International: **http://www.medhelp.org/HealthTopics/A.html**

- Open Directory Project: **http://dmoz.org/Health/Conditions_and_Diseases/**

- Yahoo.com: **http://dir.yahoo.com/Health/Diseases_and_Conditions/**

- WebMD®Health: **http://my.webmd.com/health_topics**

Finding Associations

There are several Internet directories that provide lists of medical associations with information on or resources relating to diphenhydramine. By consulting all of associations listed in this chapter, you will have nearly exhausted all sources for patient associations concerned with diphenhydramine.

The National Health Information Center (NHIC)

The National Health Information Center (NHIC) offers a free referral service to help people find organizations that provide information about diphenhydramine. For more information, see the NHIC's Web site at **http://www.health.gov/NHIC/** or contact an information specialist by calling 1-800-336-4797.

Directory of Health Organizations

The Directory of Health Organizations, provided by the National Library of Medicine Specialized Information Services, is a comprehensive source of information on associations. The Directory of Health Organizations database can be accessed via the Internet at **http://www.sis.nlm.nih.gov/Dir/DirMain.html**. It is composed of two parts: DIRLINE and Health Hotlines.

The DIRLINE database comprises some 10,000 records of organizations, research centers, and government institutes and associations that primarily focus on health and biomedicine. To access DIRLINE directly, go to the following Web site: **http://dirline.nlm.nih.gov/**. Simply type in "diphenhydramine" (or a synonym), and you will receive information on all relevant organizations listed in the database.

Health Hotlines directs you to toll-free numbers to over 300 organizations. You can access this database directly at **http://www.sis.nlm.nih.gov/hotlines/**. On this page, you are given the option to search by keyword or by browsing the subject list. When you have received your search results, click on the name of the organization for its description and contact information.

The Combined Health Information Database

Another comprehensive source of information on healthcare associations is the Combined Health Information Database. Using the "Detailed Search" option, you will need to limit your search to "Organizations" and "diphenhydramine". Type the following hyperlink into your Web browser: **http://chid.nih.gov/detail/detail.html**. To find associations, use the drop boxes at the bottom of the search page where "You may refine your search by." For publication date, select "All Years." Then, select your preferred language and the format option "Organization Resource Sheet." Type "diphenhydramine" (or synonyms) into the "For these words:" box. You should check back periodically with this database since it is updated every three months.

The National Organization for Rare Disorders, Inc.

The National Organization for Rare Disorders, Inc. has prepared a Web site that provides, at no charge, lists of associations organized by health topic. You can access this database at the following Web site: **http://www.rarediseases.org/search/orgsearch.html**. Type "diphenhydramine" (or a synonym) into the search box, and click "Submit Query."

APPENDIX C. FINDING MEDICAL LIBRARIES

Overview

In this Appendix, we show you how to quickly find a medical library in your area.

Preparation

Your local public library and medical libraries have interlibrary loan programs with the National Library of Medicine (NLM), one of the largest medical collections in the world. According to the NLM, most of the literature in the general and historical collections of the National Library of Medicine is available on interlibrary loan to any library. If you would like to access NLM medical literature, then visit a library in your area that can request the publications for you.[21]

Finding a Local Medical Library

The quickest method to locate medical libraries is to use the Internet-based directory published by the National Network of Libraries of Medicine (NN/LM). This network includes 4626 members and affiliates that provide many services to librarians, health professionals, and the public. To find a library in your area, simply visit **http://nnlm.gov/members/adv.html** or call 1-800-338-7657.

Medical Libraries in the U.S. and Canada

In addition to the NN/LM, the National Library of Medicine (NLM) lists a number of libraries with reference facilities that are open to the public. The following is the NLM's list and includes hyperlinks to each library's Web site. These Web pages can provide information on hours of operation and other restrictions. The list below is a small sample of

---

[21] Adapted from the NLM: **http://www.nlm.nih.gov/psd/cas/interlibrary.html**.

libraries recommended by the National Library of Medicine (sorted alphabetically by name of the U.S. state or Canadian province where the library is located)[22]:

- **Alabama:** Health InfoNet of Jefferson County (Jefferson County Library Cooperative, Lister Hill Library of the Health Sciences), **http://www.uab.edu/infonet/**

- **Alabama:** Richard M. Scrushy Library (American Sports Medicine Institute)

- **Arizona:** Samaritan Regional Medical Center: The Learning Center (Samaritan Health System, Phoenix, Arizona), **http://www.samaritan.edu/library/bannerlibs.htm**

- **California:** Kris Kelly Health Information Center (St. Joseph Health System, Humboldt), **http://www.humboldt1.com/~kkhic/index.html**

- **California:** Community Health Library of Los Gatos, **http://www.healthlib.org/orgresources.html**

- **California:** Consumer Health Program and Services (CHIPS) (County of Los Angeles Public Library, Los Angeles County Harbor-UCLA Medical Center Library) - Carson, CA, **http://www.colapublib.org/services/chips.html**

- **California:** Gateway Health Library (Sutter Gould Medical Foundation)

- **California:** Health Library (Stanford University Medical Center), **http://www-med.stanford.edu/healthlibrary/**

- **California:** Patient Education Resource Center - Health Information and Resources (University of California, San Francisco), **http://sfghdean.ucsf.edu/barnett/PERC/default.asp**

- **California:** Redwood Health Library (Petaluma Health Care District), **http://www.phcd.org/rdwdlib.html**

- **California:** Los Gatos PlaneTree Health Library, **http://planetreesanjose.org/**

- **California:** Sutter Resource Library (Sutter Hospitals Foundation, Sacramento), **http://suttermedicalcenter.org/library/**

- **California:** Health Sciences Libraries (University of California, Davis), **http://www.lib.ucdavis.edu/healthsci/**

- **California:** ValleyCare Health Library & Ryan Comer Cancer Resource Center (ValleyCare Health System, Pleasanton), **http://gaelnet.stmarys-ca.edu/other.libs/gbal/east/vchl.html**

- **California:** Washington Community Health Resource Library (Fremont), **http://www.healthlibrary.org/**

- **Colorado:** William V. Gervasini Memorial Library (Exempla Healthcare), **http://www.saintjosephdenver.org/yourhealth/libraries/**

- **Connecticut:** Hartford Hospital Health Science Libraries (Hartford Hospital), **http://www.harthosp.org/library/**

- **Connecticut:** Healthnet: Connecticut Consumer Health Information Center (University of Connecticut Health Center, Lyman Maynard Stowe Library), **http://library.uchc.edu/departm/hnet/**

---

[22] Abstracted from **http://www.nlm.nih.gov/medlineplus/libraries.html**.

- **Connecticut:** Waterbury Hospital Health Center Library (Waterbury Hospital, Waterbury), **http://www.waterburyhospital.com/library/consumer.shtml**

- **Delaware:** Consumer Health Library (Christiana Care Health System, Eugene du Pont Preventive Medicine & Rehabilitation Institute, Wilmington), **http://www.christianacare.org/health_guide/health_guide_pmri_health_info.cfm**

- **Delaware:** Lewis B. Flinn Library (Delaware Academy of Medicine, Wilmington), **http://www.delamed.org/chls.html**

- **Georgia:** Family Resource Library (Medical College of Georgia, Augusta), **http://cmc.mcg.edu/kids_families/fam_resources/fam_res_lib/frl.htm**

- **Georgia:** Health Resource Center (Medical Center of Central Georgia, Macon), **http://www.mccg.org/hrc/hrchome.asp**

- **Hawaii:** Hawaii Medical Library: Consumer Health Information Service (Hawaii Medical Library, Honolulu), **http://hml.org/CHIS/**

- **Idaho:** DeArmond Consumer Health Library (Kootenai Medical Center, Coeur d'Alene), **http://www.nicon.org/DeArmond/index.htm**

- **Illinois:** Health Learning Center of Northwestern Memorial Hospital (Chicago), **http://www.nmh.org/health_info/hlc.html**

- **Illinois:** Medical Library (OSF Saint Francis Medical Center, Peoria), **http://www.osfsaintfrancis.org/general/library/**

- **Kentucky:** Medical Library - Services for Patients, Families, Students & the Public (Central Baptist Hospital, Lexington), **http://www.centralbap.com/education/community/library.cfm**

- **Kentucky:** University of Kentucky - Health Information Library (Chandler Medical Center, Lexington), **http://www.mc.uky.edu/PatientEd/**

- **Louisiana:** Alton Ochsner Medical Foundation Library (Alton Ochsner Medical Foundation, New Orleans), **http://www.ochsner.org/library/**

- **Louisiana:** Louisiana State University Health Sciences Center Medical Library-Shreveport, **http://lib-sh.lsuhsc.edu/**

- **Maine:** Franklin Memorial Hospital Medical Library (Franklin Memorial Hospital, Farmington), **http://www.fchn.org/fmh/lib.htm**

- **Maine:** Gerrish-True Health Sciences Library (Central Maine Medical Center, Lewiston), **http://www.cmmc.org/library/library.html**

- **Maine:** Hadley Parrot Health Science Library (Eastern Maine Healthcare, Bangor), **http://www.emh.org/hll/hpl/guide.htm**

- **Maine:** Maine Medical Center Library (Maine Medical Center, Portland), **http://www.mmc.org/library/**

- **Maine:** Parkview Hospital (Brunswick), **http://www.parkviewhospital.org/**

- **Maine:** Southern Maine Medical Center Health Sciences Library (Southern Maine Medical Center, Biddeford), **http://www.smmc.org/services/service.php3?choice=10**

- **Maine:** Stephens Memorial Hospital's Health Information Library (Western Maine Health, Norway), **http://www.wmhcc.org/Library/**

- **Manitoba, Canada:** Consumer & Patient Health Information Service (University of Manitoba Libraries), http://www.umanitoba.ca/libraries/units/health/reference/chis.html

- **Manitoba, Canada:** J.W. Crane Memorial Library (Deer Lodge Centre, Winnipeg), http://www.deerlodge.mb.ca/crane_library/about.asp

- **Maryland:** Health Information Center at the Wheaton Regional Library (Montgomery County, Dept. of Public Libraries, Wheaton Regional Library), http://www.mont.lib.md.us/healthinfo/hic.asp

- **Massachusetts:** Baystate Medical Center Library (Baystate Health System), http://www.baystatehealth.com/1024/

- **Massachusetts:** Boston University Medical Center Alumni Medical Library (Boston University Medical Center), http://med-libwww.bu.edu/library/lib.html

- **Massachusetts:** Lowell General Hospital Health Sciences Library (Lowell General Hospital, Lowell), http://www.lowellgeneral.org/library/HomePageLinks/WWW.htm

- **Massachusetts:** Paul E. Woodard Health Sciences Library (New England Baptist Hospital, Boston), http://www.nebh.org/health_lib.asp

- **Massachusetts:** St. Luke's Hospital Health Sciences Library (St. Luke's Hospital, Southcoast Health System, New Bedford), http://www.southcoast.org/library/

- **Massachusetts:** Treadwell Library Consumer Health Reference Center (Massachusetts General Hospital), http://www.mgh.harvard.edu/library/chrcindex.html

- **Massachusetts:** UMass HealthNet (University of Massachusetts Medical School, Worchester), http://healthnet.umassmed.edu/

- **Michigan:** Botsford General Hospital Library - Consumer Health (Botsford General Hospital, Library & Internet Services), http://www.botsfordlibrary.org/consumer.htm

- **Michigan:** Helen DeRoy Medical Library (Providence Hospital and Medical Centers), http://www.providence-hospital.org/library/

- **Michigan:** Marquette General Hospital - Consumer Health Library (Marquette General Hospital, Health Information Center), http://www.mgh.org/center.html

- **Michigan:** Patient Education Resouce Center - University of Michigan Cancer Center (University of Michigan Comprehensive Cancer Center, Ann Arbor), http://www.cancer.med.umich.edu/learn/leares.htm

- **Michigan:** Sladen Library & Center for Health Information Resources - Consumer Health Information (Detroit), http://www.henryford.com/body.cfm?id=39330

- **Montana:** Center for Health Information (St. Patrick Hospital and Health Sciences Center, Missoula)

- **National:** Consumer Health Library Directory (Medical Library Association, Consumer and Patient Health Information Section), http://caphis.mlanet.org/directory/index.html

- **National:** National Network of Libraries of Medicine (National Library of Medicine) - provides library services for health professionals in the United States who do not have access to a medical library, http://nnlm.gov/

- **National:** NN/LM List of Libraries Serving the Public (National Network of Libraries of Medicine), http://nnlm.gov/members/

- **Nevada:** Health Science Library, West Charleston Library (Las Vegas-Clark County Library District, Las Vegas), **http://www.lvccld.org/special_collections/medical/index.htm**

- **New Hampshire:** Dartmouth Biomedical Libraries (Dartmouth College Library, Hanover), **http://www.dartmouth.edu/~biomed/resources.htmld/conshealth.htmld/**

- **New Jersey:** Consumer Health Library (Rahway Hospital, Rahway), **http://www.rahwayhospital.com/library.htm**

- **New Jersey:** Dr. Walter Phillips Health Sciences Library (Englewood Hospital and Medical Center, Englewood), **http://www.englewoodhospital.com/links/index.htm**

- **New Jersey:** Meland Foundation (Englewood Hospital and Medical Center, Englewood), **http://www.geocities.com/ResearchTriangle/9360/**

- **New York:** Choices in Health Information (New York Public Library) - NLM Consumer Pilot Project participant, **http://www.nypl.org/branch/health/links.html**

- **New York:** Health Information Center (Upstate Medical University, State University of New York, Syracuse), **http://www.upstate.edu/library/hic/**

- **New York:** Health Sciences Library (Long Island Jewish Medical Center, New Hyde Park), **http://www.lij.edu/library/library.html**

- **New York:** ViaHealth Medical Library (Rochester General Hospital), **http://www.nyam.org/library/**

- **Ohio:** Consumer Health Library (Akron General Medical Center, Medical & Consumer Health Library), **http://www.akrongeneral.org/hwlibrary.htm**

- **Oklahoma:** The Health Information Center at Saint Francis Hospital (Saint Francis Health System, Tulsa), **http://www.sfh-tulsa.com/services/healthinfo.asp**

- **Oregon:** Planetree Health Resource Center (Mid-Columbia Medical Center, The Dalles), **http://www.mcmc.net/phrc/**

- **Pennsylvania:** Community Health Information Library (Milton S. Hershey Medical Center, Hershey), **http://www.hmc.psu.edu/commhealth/**

- **Pennsylvania:** Community Health Resource Library (Geisinger Medical Center, Danville), **http://www.geisinger.edu/education/commlib.shtml**

- **Pennsylvania:** HealthInfo Library (Moses Taylor Hospital, Scranton), **http://www.mth.org/healthwellness.html**

- **Pennsylvania:** Hopwood Library (University of Pittsburgh, Health Sciences Library System, Pittsburgh), **http://www.hsls.pitt.edu/guides/chi/hopwood/index_html**

- **Pennsylvania:** Koop Community Health Information Center (College of Physicians of Philadelphia), **http://www.collphyphil.org/kooppg1.shtml**

- **Pennsylvania:** Learning Resources Center - Medical Library (Susquehanna Health System, Williamsport), **http://www.shscares.org/services/lrc/index.asp**

- **Pennsylvania:** Medical Library (UPMC Health System, Pittsburgh), **http://www.upmc.edu/passavant/library.htm**

- **Quebec, Canada:** Medical Library (Montreal General Hospital), **http://www.mghlib.mcgill.ca/**

- **South Dakota:** Rapid City Regional Hospital Medical Library (Rapid City Regional Hospital), **http://www.rcrh.org/Services/Library/Default.asp**

- **Texas:** Houston HealthWays (Houston Academy of Medicine-Texas Medical Center Library), **http://hhw.library.tmc.edu/**

- **Washington:** Community Health Library (Kittitas Valley Community Hospital), **http://www.kvch.com/**

- **Washington:** Southwest Washington Medical Center Library (Southwest Washington Medical Center, Vancouver), **http://www.swmedicalcenter.com/body.cfm?id=72**

ONLINE GLOSSARIES

The Internet provides access to a number of free-to-use medical dictionaries. The National Library of Medicine has compiled the following list of online dictionaries:

- ADAM Medical Encyclopedia (A.D.A.M., Inc.), comprehensive medical reference: **http://www.nlm.nih.gov/medlineplus/encyclopedia.html**

- MedicineNet.com Medical Dictionary (MedicineNet, Inc.): **http://www.medterms.com/Script/Main/hp.asp**

- Merriam-Webster Medical Dictionary (Inteli-Health, Inc.): **http://www.intelihealth.com/IH/**

- Multilingual Glossary of Technical and Popular Medical Terms in Eight European Languages (European Commission) - Danish, Dutch, English, French, German, Italian, Portuguese, and Spanish: **http://allserv.rug.ac.be/~rvdstich/eugloss/welcome.html**

- On-line Medical Dictionary (CancerWEB): **http://cancerweb.ncl.ac.uk/omd/**

- Rare Diseases Terms (Office of Rare Diseases): **http://ord.aspensys.com/asp/diseases/diseases.asp**

- Technology Glossary (National Library of Medicine) - Health Care Technology: **http://www.nlm.nih.gov/nichsr/ta101/ta10108.htm**

Beyond these, MEDLINEplus contains a very patient-friendly encyclopedia covering every aspect of medicine (licensed from A.D.A.M., Inc.). The ADAM Medical Encyclopedia can be accessed at **http://www.nlm.nih.gov/medlineplus/encyclopedia.html**. ADAM is also available on commercial Web sites such as drkoop.com (**http://www.drkoop.com/**) and Web MD (**http://my.webmd.com/adam/asset/adam_disease_articles/a_to_z/a**). The NIH suggests the following Web sites in the ADAM Medical Encyclopedia when searching for information on diphenhydramine:

- **Basic Guidelines for Diphenhydramine**

    Diphenhydramine hydrochloride overdose
    Web site: http://www.nlm.nih.gov/medlineplus/ency/article/002636.htm

- **Signs & Symptoms for Diphenhydramine**

    Agitation
    Web site: http://www.nlm.nih.gov/medlineplus/ency/article/003212.htm

    Blurred vision
    Web site: http://www.nlm.nih.gov/medlineplus/ency/article/003029.htm

    Coma
    Web site: http://www.nlm.nih.gov/medlineplus/ency/article/003202.htm

    Confusion
    Web site: http://www.nlm.nih.gov/medlineplus/ency/article/003205.htm

Convulsions
Web site: http://www.nlm.nih.gov/medlineplus/ency/article/003200.htm

Diarrhea
Web site: http://www.nlm.nih.gov/medlineplus/ency/article/003126.htm

Drowsiness
Web site: http://www.nlm.nih.gov/medlineplus/ency/article/003208.htm

Emesis
Web site: http://www.nlm.nih.gov/medlineplus/ency/article/003117.htm

Headache
Web site: http://www.nlm.nih.gov/medlineplus/ency/article/003024.htm

Nausea and/or vomiting
Web site: http://www.nlm.nih.gov/medlineplus/ency/article/003117.htm

Rapid breathing
Web site: http://www.nlm.nih.gov/medlineplus/ency/article/003071.htm

Rash
Web site: http://www.nlm.nih.gov/medlineplus/ency/article/003220.htm

Ringing in the ears
Web site: http://www.nlm.nih.gov/medlineplus/ency/article/003043.htm

Stomach pain
Web site: http://www.nlm.nih.gov/medlineplus/ency/article/003120.htm

Unsteadiness
Web site: http://www.nlm.nih.gov/medlineplus/ency/article/003199.htm

Vomiting
Web site: http://www.nlm.nih.gov/medlineplus/ency/article/003117.htm

- **Diagnostics and Tests for Diphenhydramine**

  Gastric lavage
  Web site: http://www.nlm.nih.gov/medlineplus/ency/article/003882.htm

- **Background Topics for Diphenhydramine**

  Labored breathing
  Web site: http://www.nlm.nih.gov/medlineplus/ency/article/000007.htm

  Respiratory
  Web site: http://www.nlm.nih.gov/medlineplus/ency/article/002290.htm

  Unconscious
  Web site: http://www.nlm.nih.gov/medlineplus/ency/article/000022.htm

Online Dictionary Directories

The following are additional online directories compiled by the National Library of Medicine, including a number of specialized medical dictionaries:

- Medical Dictionaries: Medical & Biological (World Health Organization):
  http://www.who.int/hlt/virtuallibrary/English/diction.htm#Medical

- MEL-Michigan Electronic Library List of Online Health and Medical Dictionaries (Michigan Electronic Library): **http://mel.lib.mi.us/health/health-dictionaries.html**

- Patient Education: Glossaries (DMOZ Open Directory Project):
  http://dmoz.org/Health/Education/Patient_Education/Glossaries/

- Web of Online Dictionaries (Bucknell University):
  http://www.yourdictionary.com/diction5.html#medicine

DIPHENHYDRAMINE DICTIONARY

The definitions below are derived from official public sources, including the National Institutes of Health [NIH] and the European Union [EU].

Abdominal: Having to do with the abdomen, which is the part of the body between the chest and the hips that contains the pancreas, stomach, intestines, liver, gallbladder, and other organs. [NIH]

Abdominal Pain: Sensation of discomfort, distress, or agony in the abdominal region. [NIH]

Acantholysis: Separation of the prickle cells of the stratum spinosum of the epidermis, resulting in atrophy of the prickle cell layer. It is seen in diseases such as pemphigus vulgaris (see pemphigus) and keratosis follicularis. [NIH]

Acetaminophen: Analgesic antipyretic derivative of acetanilide. It has weak anti-inflammatory properties and is used as a common analgesic, but may cause liver, blood cell, and kidney damage. [NIH]

Acetylcholine: A neurotransmitter. Acetylcholine in vertebrates is the major transmitter at neuromuscular junctions, autonomic ganglia, parasympathetic effector junctions, a subset of sympathetic effector junctions, and at many sites in the central nervous system. It is generally not used as an administered drug because it is broken down very rapidly by cholinesterases, but it is useful in some ophthalmological applications. [NIH]

Activities of Daily Living: The performance of the basic activities of self care, such as dressing, ambulation, eating, etc., in rehabilitation. [NIH]

Acute renal: A condition in which the kidneys suddenly stop working. In most cases, kidneys can recover from almost complete loss of function. [NIH]

Adaptation: 1. The adjustment of an organism to its environment, or the process by which it enhances such fitness. 2. The normal ability of the eye to adjust itself to variations in the intensity of light; the adjustment to such variations. 3. The decline in the frequency of firing of a neuron, particularly of a receptor, under conditions of constant stimulation. 4. In dentistry, (a) the proper fitting of a denture, (b) the degree of proximity and interlocking of restorative material to a tooth preparation, (c) the exact adjustment of bands to teeth. 5. In microbiology, the adjustment of bacterial physiology to a new environment. [EU]

Adenosine: A nucleoside that is composed of adenine and d-ribose. Adenosine or adenosine derivatives play many important biological roles in addition to being components of DNA and RNA. Adenosine itself is a neurotransmitter. [NIH]

Adjunctive Therapy: Another treatment used together with the primary treatment. Its purpose is to assist the primary treatment. [NIH]

Adjuvant: A substance which aids another, such as an auxiliary remedy; in immunology, nonspecific stimulator (e.g., BCG vaccine) of the immune response. [EU]

Adrenal Medulla: The inner part of the adrenal gland; it synthesizes, stores and releases catecholamines. [NIH]

Adrenergic: Activated by, characteristic of, or secreting epinephrine or substances with similar activity; the term is applied to those nerve fibres that liberate norepinephrine at a synapse when a nerve impulse passes, i.e., the sympathetic fibres. [EU]

Adrenergic Agonists: Drugs that bind to and activate adrenergic receptors. [NIH]

Adsorption: The condensation of gases, liquids, or dissolved substances on the surfaces of solids. It includes adsorptive phenomena of bacteria and viruses as well as of tissues treated with exogenous drugs and chemicals. [NIH]

Adsorptive: It captures volatile compounds by binding them to agents such as activated carbon or adsorptive resins. [NIH]

Adverse Effect: An unwanted side effect of treatment. [NIH]

Aerosol: A solution of a drug which can be atomized into a fine mist for inhalation therapy. [EU]

Affinity: 1. Inherent likeness or relationship. 2. A special attraction for a specific element, organ, or structure. 3. Chemical affinity; the force that binds atoms in molecules; the tendency of substances to combine by chemical reaction. 4. The strength of noncovalent chemical binding between two substances as measured by the dissociation constant of the complex. 5. In immunology, a thermodynamic expression of the strength of interaction between a single antigen-binding site and a single antigenic determinant (and thus of the stereochemical compatibility between them), most accurately applied to interactions among simple, uniform antigenic determinants such as haptens. Expressed as the association constant (K litres mole -1), which, owing to the heterogeneity of affinities in a population of antibody molecules of a given specificity, actually represents an average value (mean intrinsic association constant). 6. The reciprocal of the dissociation constant. [EU]

Agarose: A polysaccharide complex, free of nitrogen and prepared from agar-agar which is produced by certain seaweeds (red algae). It dissolves in warm water to form a viscid solution. [NIH]

Agonist: In anatomy, a prime mover. In pharmacology, a drug that has affinity for and stimulates physiologic activity at cell receptors normally stimulated by naturally occurring substances. [EU]

Airway: A device for securing unobstructed passage of air into and out of the lungs during general anesthesia. [NIH]

Akathisia: 1. A condition of motor restlessness in which there is a feeling of muscular quivering, an urge to move about constantly, and an inability to sit still, a common extrapyramidal side effect of neuroleptic drugs. 2. An inability to sit down because of intense anxiety at the thought of doing so. [EU]

Albumin: 1. Any protein that is soluble in water and moderately concentrated salt solutions and is coagulable by heat. 2. Serum albumin; the major plasma protein (approximately 60 per cent of the total), which is responsible for much of the plasma colloidal osmotic pressure and serves as a transport protein carrying large organic anions, such as fatty acids, bilirubin, and many drugs, and also carrying certain hormones, such as cortisol and thyroxine, when their specific binding globulins are saturated. Albumin is synthesized in the liver. Low serum levels occur in protein malnutrition, active inflammation and serious hepatic and renal disease. [EU]

Alertness: A state of readiness to detect and respond to certain specified small changes occurring at random intervals in the environment. [NIH]

Algorithms: A procedure consisting of a sequence of algebraic formulas and/or logical steps to calculate or determine a given task. [NIH]

Alkaline: Having the reactions of an alkali. [EU]

Alkaloid: A member of a large group of chemicals that are made by plants and have nitrogen in them. Some alkaloids have been shown to work against cancer. [NIH]

Allergen: An antigenic substance capable of producing immediate-type hypersensitivity (allergy). [EU]

Allergic Rhinitis: Inflammation of the nasal mucous membrane associated with hay fever; fits may be provoked by substances in the working environment. [NIH]

Allylamine: Possesses an unusual and selective cytotoxicity for vascular smooth muscle cells in dogs and rats. Useful for experiments dealing with arterial injury, myocardial fibrosis or cardiac decompensation. [NIH]

Aloe: A genus of the family Liliaceae containing anthraquinone glycosides such as aloin-emodin or aloe-emodin (emodin). [NIH]

Alopecia: Absence of hair from areas where it is normally present. [NIH]

Alpha-1: A protein with the property of inactivating proteolytic enzymes such as leucocyte collagenase and elastase. [NIH]

Alprenolol: 1-((1-Methylethyl)amino)-3-(2-(2-propenyl)phenoxy)-2-propanol. Adrenergic beta-blocker used as an antihypertensive, anti-anginal, and anti-arrhythmic agent. [NIH]

Alternative medicine: Practices not generally recognized by the medical community as standard or conventional medical approaches and used instead of standard treatments. Alternative medicine includes the taking of dietary supplements, megadose vitamins, and herbal preparations; the drinking of special teas; and practices such as massage therapy, magnet therapy, spiritual healing, and meditation. [NIH]

Aluminum: A metallic element that has the atomic number 13, atomic symbol Al, and atomic weight 26.98. [NIH]

Alveoli: Tiny air sacs at the end of the bronchioles in the lungs. [NIH]

Amine: An organic compound containing nitrogen; any member of a group of chemical compounds formed from ammonia by replacement of one or more of the hydrogen atoms by organic (hydrocarbon) radicals. The amines are distinguished as primary, secondary, and tertiary, according to whether one, two, or three hydrogen atoms are replaced. The amines include allylamine, amylamine, ethylamine, methylamine, phenylamine, propylamine, and many other compounds. [EU]

Amino Acids: Organic compounds that generally contain an amino (-NH2) and a carboxyl (-COOH) group. Twenty alpha-amino acids are the subunits which are polymerized to form proteins. [NIH]

Amino Acids: Organic compounds that generally contain an amino (-NH2) and a carboxyl (-COOH) group. Twenty alpha-amino acids are the subunits which are polymerized to form proteins. [NIH]

Amitriptyline: Tricyclic antidepressant with anticholinergic and sedative properties. It appears to prevent the re-uptake of norepinephrine and serotonin at nerve terminals, thus potentiating the action of these neurotransmitters. Amitriptyline also appears to antaganize cholinergic and alpha-1 adrenergic responses to bioactive amines. [NIH]

Ammonia: A colorless alkaline gas. It is formed in the body during decomposition of organic materials during a large number of metabolically important reactions. [NIH]

Amphetamines: Analogs or derivatives of amphetamine. Many are sympathomimetics and central nervous system stimulators causing excitation, vasopression, bronchodilation, and to varying degrees, anorexia, analepsis, nasal decongestion, and some smooth muscle relaxation. [NIH]

Analgesic: An agent that alleviates pain without causing loss of consciousness. [EU]

Analog: In chemistry, a substance that is similar, but not identical, to another. [NIH]

Anaphylactic: Pertaining to anaphylaxis. [EU]

Anaphylaxis: An acute hypersensitivity reaction due to exposure to a previously encountered antigen. The reaction may include rapidly progressing urticaria, respiratory distress, vascular collapse, systemic shock, and death. [NIH]

Anatomical: Pertaining to anatomy, or to the structure of the organism. [EU]

Anesthesia: A state characterized by loss of feeling or sensation. This depression of nerve function is usually the result of pharmacologic action and is induced to allow performance of surgery or other painful procedures. [NIH]

Anesthetics: Agents that are capable of inducing a total or partial loss of sensation, especially tactile sensation and pain. They may act to induce general anesthesia, in which an unconscious state is achieved, or may act locally to induce numbness or lack of sensation at a targeted site. [NIH]

Angina: Chest pain that originates in the heart. [NIH]

Angina Pectoris: The symptom of paroxysmal pain consequent to myocardial ischemia usually of distinctive character, location and radiation, and provoked by a transient stressful situation during which the oxygen requirements of the myocardium exceed the capacity of the coronary circulation to supply it. [NIH]

Anionic: Pertaining to or containing an anion. [EU]

Anions: Negatively charged atoms, radicals or groups of atoms which travel to the anode or positive pole during electrolysis. [NIH]

Antagonism: Interference with, or inhibition of, the growth of a living organism by another living organism, due either to creation of unfavorable conditions (e. g. exhaustion of food supplies) or to production of a specific antibiotic substance (e. g. penicillin). [NIH]

Antazoline: An antagonist of histamine H1 receptors. [NIH]

Anthelmintic: An agent that is destructive to worms. [EU]

Antiallergic: Counteracting allergy or allergic conditions. [EU]

Anti-Anxiety Agents: Agents that alleviate anxiety, tension, and neurotic symptoms, promote sedation, and have a calming effect without affecting clarity of consciousness or neurologic conditions. Some are also effective as anticonvulsants, muscle relaxants, or anesthesia adjuvants. Adrenergic beta-antagonists are commonly used in the symptomatic treatment of anxiety but are not included here. [NIH]

Antibacterial: A substance that destroys bacteria or suppresses their growth or reproduction. [EU]

Antibiotic: A drug used to treat infections caused by bacteria and other microorganisms. [NIH]

Antibiotic Prophylaxis: Use of antibiotics before, during, or after a diagnostic, therapeutic, or surgical procedure to prevent infectious complications. [NIH]

Antibody: A type of protein made by certain white blood cells in response to a foreign substance (antigen). Each antibody can bind to only a specific antigen. The purpose of this binding is to help destroy the antigen. Antibodies can work in several ways, depending on the nature of the antigen. Some antibodies destroy antigens directly. Others make it easier for white blood cells to destroy the antigen. [NIH]

Anticholinergic: An agent that blocks the parasympathetic nerves. Called also parasympatholytic. [EU]

Anticonvulsant: An agent that prevents or relieves convulsions. [EU]

Antidepressant: A drug used to treat depression. [NIH]

Antidopaminergic: Preventing or counteracting (the effects of) dopamine. [EU]

Antiemetic: An agent that prevents or alleviates nausea and vomiting. Also antinauseant. [EU]

Antifungal: Destructive to fungi, or suppressing their reproduction or growth; effective against fungal infections. [EU]

Antigen: Any substance which is capable, under appropriate conditions, of inducing a specific immune response and of reacting with the products of that response, that is, with specific antibody or specifically sensitized T-lymphocytes, or both. Antigens may be soluble substances, such as toxins and foreign proteins, or particulate, such as bacteria and tissue cells; however, only the portion of the protein or polysaccharide molecule known as the antigenic determinant (q.v.) combines with antibody or a specific receptor on a lymphocyte. Abbreviated Ag. [EU]

Antihistamine: A drug that counteracts the action of histamine. The antihistamines are of two types. The conventional ones, as those used in allergies, block the H1 histamine receptors, whereas the others block the H2 receptors. Called also antihistaminic. [EU]

Anti-infective: An agent that so acts. [EU]

Anti-inflammatory: Having to do with reducing inflammation. [NIH]

Anti-Inflammatory Agents: Substances that reduce or suppress inflammation. [NIH]

Antimetabolite: A chemical that is very similar to one required in a normal biochemical reaction in cells. Antimetabolites can stop or slow down the reaction. [NIH]

Antimicrobial: Killing microorganisms, or suppressing their multiplication or growth. [EU]

Antimycotic: Suppressing the growth of fungi. [EU]

Antineoplastic: Inhibiting or preventing the development of neoplasms, checking the maturation and proliferation of malignant cells. [EU]

Antipsychotic: Effective in the treatment of psychosis. Antipsychotic drugs (called also neuroleptic drugs and major tranquilizers) are a chemically diverse (including phenothiazines, thioxanthenes, butyrophenones, dibenzoxazepines, dibenzodiazepines, and diphenylbutylpiperidines) but pharmacologically similar class of drugs used to treat schizophrenic, paranoid, schizoaffective, and other psychotic disorders; acute delirium and dementia, and manic episodes (during induction of lithium therapy); to control the movement disorders associated with Huntington's chorea, Gilles de la Tourette's syndrome, and ballismus; and to treat intractable hiccups and severe nausea and vomiting. Antipsychotic agents bind to dopamine, histamine, muscarinic cholinergic, a-adrenergic, and serotonin receptors. Blockade of dopaminergic transmission in various areas is thought to be responsible for their major effects : antipsychotic action by blockade in the mesolimbic and mesocortical areas; extrapyramidal side effects (dystonia, akathisia, parkinsonism, and tardive dyskinesia) by blockade in the basal ganglia; and antiemetic effects by blockade in the chemoreceptor trigger zone of the medulla. Sedation and autonomic side effects (orthostatic hypotension, blurred vision, dry mouth, nasal congestion and constipation) are caused by blockade of histamine, cholinergic, and adrenergic receptors. [EU]

Antipyretic: An agent that relieves or reduces fever. Called also antifebrile, antithermic and febrifuge. [EU]

Antispasmodic: An agent that relieves spasm. [EU]

Antitussive: An agent that relieves or prevents cough. [EU]

Anus: The opening of the rectum to the outside of the body. [NIH]

Anxiety: Persistent feeling of dread, apprehension, and impending disaster. [NIH]

Anxiolytic: An anxiolytic or antianxiety agent. [EU]

Apathy: Lack of feeling or emotion; indifference. [EU]

Apocrine Glands: Large, branched, specialized sweat glands that empty into the upper portion of a hair follicle instead of directly onto the skin. [NIH]

Aqueous: Having to do with water. [NIH]

Arterial: Pertaining to an artery or to the arteries. [EU]

Arterioles: The smallest divisions of the arteries located between the muscular arteries and the capillaries. [NIH]

Articular: Of or pertaining to a joint. [EU]

Aspartate: A synthetic amino acid. [NIH]

Asphyxia: A pathological condition caused by lack of oxygen, manifested in impending or actual cessation of life. [NIH]

Aspiration: The act of inhaling. [NIH]

Aspirin: A drug that reduces pain, fever, inflammation, and blood clotting. Aspirin belongs to the family of drugs called nonsteroidal anti-inflammatory agents. It is also being studied in cancer prevention. [NIH]

Assay: Determination of the amount of a particular constituent of a mixture, or of the biological or pharmacological potency of a drug. [EU]

Astringent: Causing contraction, usually locally after topical application. [EU]

Asymptomatic: Having no signs or symptoms of disease. [NIH]

Ataxia: Impairment of the ability to perform smoothly coordinated voluntary movements. This condition may affect the limbs, trunk, eyes, pharnyx, larnyx, and other structures. Ataxia may result from impaired sensory or motor function. Sensory ataxia may result from posterior column injury or peripheral nerve diseases. Motor ataxia may be associated with cerebellar diseases; cerebral cortex diseases; thalamic diseases; basal ganglia diseases; injury to the red nucleus; and other conditions. [NIH]

Atrophy: Decrease in the size of a cell, tissue, organ, or multiple organs, associated with a variety of pathological conditions such as abnormal cellular changes, ischemia, malnutrition, or hormonal changes. [NIH]

Atropine: A toxic alkaloid, originally from Atropa belladonna, but found in other plants, mainly Solanaceae. [NIH]

Auditory: Pertaining to the sense of hearing. [EU]

Automobile Driving: The effect of environmental or physiological factors on the driver and driving ability. Included are driving fatigue, and the effect of drugs, disease, and physical disabilities on driving. [NIH]

Autonomic Nervous System: The enteric, parasympathetic, and sympathetic nervous systems taken together. Generally speaking, the autonomic nervous system regulates the internal environment during both peaceful activity and physical or emotional stress. Autonomic activity is controlled and integrated by the central nervous system, especially the hypothalamus and the solitary nucleus, which receive information relayed from visceral afferents; these and related central and sensory structures are sometimes (but not here) considered to be part of the autonomic nervous system itself. [NIH]

Axillary: Pertaining to the armpit area, including the lymph nodes that are located there. [NIH]

Back Pain: Acute or chronic pain located in the posterior regions of the trunk, including the thoracic, lumbar, sacral, or adjacent regions. [NIH]

Bacteria: Unicellular prokaryotic microorganisms which generally possess rigid cell walls, multiply by cell division, and exhibit three principal forms: round or coccal, rodlike or bacillary, and spiral or spirochetal. [NIH]

Bacterial Infections: Infections by bacteria, general or unspecified. [NIH]

Bactericidal: Substance lethal to bacteria; substance capable of killing bacteria. [NIH]

Bacterium: Microscopic organism which may have a spherical, rod-like, or spiral unicellular or non-cellular body. Bacteria usually reproduce through asexual processes. [NIH]

Barbiturate: A drug with sedative and hypnotic effects. Barbiturates have been used as sedatives and anesthetics, and they have been used to treat the convulsions associated with epilepsy. [NIH]

Basal cells: Small, round cells found in the lower part (or base) of the epidermis, the outer layer of the skin. [NIH]

Basal Ganglia: Large subcortical nuclear masses derived from the telencephalon and located in the basal regions of the cerebral hemispheres. [NIH]

Basal Ganglia Diseases: Diseases of the basal ganglia including the putamen; globus pallidus; claustrum; amygdala; and caudate nucleus. Dyskinesias (most notably involuntary movements and alterations of the rate of movement) represent the primary clinical manifestations of these disorders. Common etiologies include cerebrovascular disease; neurodegenerative diseases; and craniocerebral trauma. [NIH]

Base: In chemistry, the nonacid part of a salt; a substance that combines with acids to form salts; a substance that dissociates to give hydroxide ions in aqueous solutions; a substance whose molecule or ion can combine with a proton (hydrogen ion); a substance capable of donating a pair of electrons (to an acid) for the formation of a coordinate covalent bond. [EU]

Belladonna: A species of very poisonous Solanaceous plants yielding atropine (hyoscyamine), scopolamine, and other belladonna alkaloids, used to block the muscarinic autonomic nervous system. [NIH]

Benactyzine: A centrally acting muscarinic antagonist. Benactyzine has been used in the treatment of depression and is used in research to investigate the role of cholinergic systems on behavior. [NIH]

Benign: Not cancerous; does not invade nearby tissue or spread to other parts of the body. [NIH]

Benzodiazepines: A two-ring heterocyclic compound consisting of a benzene ring fused to a diazepine ring. Permitted is any degree of hydrogenation, any substituents and any H-isomer. [NIH]

Benztropine: A centrally active muscarinic antagonist that has been used in the symptomatic treatment of Parkinson's disease. Benztropine also inhibits the uptake of dopamine. [NIH]

Benzyl Alcohol: A colorless liquid with a sharp burning taste and slight odor. It is used as a local anesthetic and to reduce pain associated with lidocaine injection. Also, it is used in the manufacture of other benzyl compounds, as a pharmaceutic aid, and in perfumery and flavoring. [NIH]

Bile: An emulsifying agent produced in the liver and secreted into the duodenum. Its composition includes bile acids and salts, cholesterol, and electrolytes. It aids digestion of fats in the duodenum. [NIH]

Bilirubin: A bile pigment that is a degradation product of heme. [NIH]

Biochemical: Relating to biochemistry; characterized by, produced by, or involving chemical reactions in living organisms. [EU]

Biotechnology: Body of knowledge related to the use of organisms, cells or cell-derived constituents for the purpose of developing products which are technically, scientifically and clinically useful. Alteration of biologic function at the molecular level (i.e., genetic engineering) is a central focus; laboratory methods used include transfection and cloning technologies, sequence and structure analysis algorithms, computer databases, and gene and protein structure function analysis and prediction. [NIH]

Biperiden: A muscarinic antagonist that has effects in both the central and peripheral nervous systems. It has been used in the treatment of arteriosclerotic, idiopathic, and postencephalitic parkinsonism. It has also been used to alleviate extrapyramidal symptoms induced by phenothiazine derivatives and reserpine. [NIH]

Bladder: The organ that stores urine. [NIH]

Blister: Visible accumulations of fluid within or beneath the epidermis. [NIH]

Bloating: Fullness or swelling in the abdomen that often occurs after meals. [NIH]

Blood Coagulation: The process of the interaction of blood coagulation factors that results in an insoluble fibrin clot. [NIH]

Blood Platelets: Non-nucleated disk-shaped cells formed in the megakaryocyte and found in the blood of all mammals. They are mainly involved in blood coagulation. [NIH]

Blood pressure: The pressure of blood against the walls of a blood vessel or heart chamber. Unless there is reference to another location, such as the pulmonary artery or one of the heart chambers, it refers to the pressure in the systemic arteries, as measured, for example, in the forearm. [NIH]

Blood vessel: A tube in the body through which blood circulates. Blood vessels include a network of arteries, arterioles, capillaries, venules, and veins. [NIH]

Blood-Brain Barrier: Specialized non-fenestrated tightly-joined endothelial cells (tight junctions) that form a transport barrier for certain substances between the cerebral capillaries and the brain tissue. [NIH]

Body Fluids: Liquid components of living organisms. [NIH]

Body Regions: Anatomical areas of the body. [NIH]

Bone Marrow: The soft tissue filling the cavities of bones. Bone marrow exists in two types, yellow and red. Yellow marrow is found in the large cavities of large bones and consists mostly of fat cells and a few primitive blood cells. Red marrow is a hematopoietic tissue and is the site of production of erythrocytes and granular leukocytes. Bone marrow is made up of a framework of connective tissue containing branching fibers with the frame being filled with marrow cells. [NIH]

Bowel: The long tube-shaped organ in the abdomen that completes the process of digestion. There is both a small and a large bowel. Also called the intestine. [NIH]

Bowel Movement: Body wastes passed through the rectum and anus. [NIH]

Broad-spectrum: Effective against a wide range of microorganisms; said of an antibiotic. [EU]

Bronchi: The larger air passages of the lungs arising from the terminal bifurcation of the trachea. [NIH]

Bronchial: Pertaining to one or more bronchi. [EU]

Bronchial Hyperreactivity: Tendency of the smooth muscle of the tracheobronchial tree to contract more intensely in response to a given stimulus than it does in the response seen in normal individuals. This condition is present in virtually all symptomatic patients with asthma. The most prominent manifestation of this smooth muscle contraction is a decrease in airway caliber that can be readily measured in the pulmonary function laboratory. [NIH]

Bronchiseptica: A small, gram-negative, motile bacillus. A normal inhabitant of the respiratory tract in man, dogs, and pigs, but is also associated with canine infectious tracheobronchitis and atrophic rhinitis in pigs. [NIH]

Bronchodilator: A drug that relaxes the smooth muscles in the constricted airway. [NIH]

Bulking Agents: Laxatives that make bowel movements soft and easy to pass. [NIH]

Bupivacaine: A widely used local anesthetic agent. [NIH]

Butorphanol: A synthetic morphinan analgesic with narcotic antagonist action. It is used in the management of severe pain. [NIH]

Caffeine: A methylxanthine naturally occurring in some beverages and also used as a pharmacological agent. Caffeine's most notable pharmacological effect is as a central nervous system stimulant, increasing alertness and producing agitation. It also relaxes smooth muscle, stimulates cardiac muscle, stimulates diuresis, and appears to be useful in the treatment of some types of headache. Several cellular actions of caffeine have been observed, but it is not entirely clear how each contributes to its pharmacological profile. Among the most important are inhibition of cyclic nucleotide phosphodiesterases, antagonism of adenosine receptors, and modulation of intracellular calcium handling. [NIH]

Calcium: A basic element found in nearly all organized tissues. It is a member of the alkaline earth family of metals with the atomic symbol Ca, atomic number 20, and atomic weight 40. Calcium is the most abundant mineral in the body and combines with phosphorus to form calcium phosphate in the bones and teeth. It is essential for the normal functioning of nerves and muscles and plays a role in blood coagulation (as factor IV) and in many enzymatic processes. [NIH]

Calcium Channel Blockers: A class of drugs that act by selective inhibition of calcium influx through cell membranes or on the release and binding of calcium in intracellular pools. Since they are inducers of vascular and other smooth muscle relaxation, they are used in the drug therapy of hypertension and cerebrovascular spasms, as myocardial protective agents, and in the relaxation of uterine spasms. [NIH]

Capillary: Any one of the minute vessels that connect the arterioles and venules, forming a network in nearly all parts of the body. Their walls act as semipermeable membranes for the interchange of various substances, including fluids, between the blood and tissue fluid; called also vas capillare. [EU]

Capsaicin: Cytotoxic alkaloid from various species of Capsicum (pepper, paprika), of the Solanaceae. [NIH]

Capsules: Hard or soft soluble containers used for the oral administration of medicine. [NIH]

Carbamazepine: An anticonvulsant used to control grand mal and psychomotor or focal seizures. Its mode of action is not fully understood, but some of its actions resemble those of phenytoin; although there is little chemical resemblance between the two compounds, their three-dimensional structure is similar. [NIH]

Carbohydrate: An aldehyde or ketone derivative of a polyhydric alcohol, particularly of the pentahydric and hexahydric alcohols. They are so named because the hydrogen and oxygen are usually in the proportion to form water, $(CH_2O)n$. The most important carbohydrates are the starches, sugars, celluloses, and gums. They are classified into mono-, di-, tri-, poly- and heterosaccharides. [EU]

Carbonate Dehydratase: A zinc-containing enzyme of erythrocytes with molecular weight of 30 kD. It is among the most active of known enzymes and catalyzes the reversible hydration of carbon dioxide, which is significant in the transport of CO_2 from the tissues to the lungs. The enzyme is inhibited by acetazolamide. EC 4.2.1.1. [NIH]

Carbonic Anhydrase Inhibitors: A class of compounds that reduces the secretion of H+ ions by the proximal kidney tubule through inhibition of carbonic anhydrase (carbonate dehydratase). [NIH]

Carcinogenesis: The process by which normal cells are transformed into cancer cells. [NIH]

Cardiac: Having to do with the heart. [NIH]

Cardiac catheterization: A procedure in which a thin, hollow tube is inserted into a blood vessel. The tube is then advanced through the vessel into the heart, enabling a physician to study the heart and its pumping activity. [NIH]

Case report: A detailed report of the diagnosis, treatment, and follow-up of an individual patient. Case reports also contain some demographic information about the patient (for example, age, gender, ethnic origin). [NIH]

Case series: A group or series of case reports involving patients who were given similar treatment. Reports of case series usually contain detailed information about the individual patients. This includes demographic information (for example, age, gender, ethnic origin) and information on diagnosis, treatment, response to treatment, and follow-up after treatment. [NIH]

Castor Oil: Oil obtained from seeds of Ricinus communis that is used as a cathartic and as a plasticizer. [NIH]

Catheterization: Use or insertion of a tubular device into a duct, blood vessel, hollow organ, or body cavity for injecting or withdrawing fluids for diagnostic or therapeutic purposes. It differs from intubation in that the tube here is used to restore or maintain patency in obstructions. [NIH]

Cations: Postively charged atoms, radicals or groups of atoms which travel to the cathode or negative pole during electrolysis. [NIH]

Cell: The individual unit that makes up all of the tissues of the body. All living things are made up of one or more cells. [NIH]

Cell Cycle: The complex series of phenomena, occurring between the end of one cell division and the end of the next, by which cellular material is divided between daughter cells. [NIH]

Cell Division: The fission of a cell. [NIH]

Cell membrane: Cell membrane = plasma membrane. The structure enveloping a cell, enclosing the cytoplasm, and forming a selective permeability barrier; it consists of lipids, proteins, and some carbohydrates, the lipids thought to form a bilayer in which integral proteins are embedded to varying degrees. [EU]

Central Nervous System: The main information-processing organs of the nervous system, consisting of the brain, spinal cord, and meninges. [NIH]

Central Nervous System Infections: Pathogenic infections of the brain, spinal cord, and meninges. DNA virus infections; RNA virus infections; bacterial infections; mycoplasma infections; Spirochaetales infections; fungal infections; protozoan infections; helminthiasis; and prion diseases may involve the central nervous system as a primary or secondary process. [NIH]

Cerebellar: Pertaining to the cerebellum. [EU]

Cerebral: Of or pertaining of the cerebrum or the brain. [EU]

Cerebral Cortex: The thin layer of gray matter on the surface of the cerebral hemisphere that develops from the telencephalon and folds into gyri. It reaches its highest development in man and is responsible for intellectual faculties and higher mental functions. [NIH]

Cerebrovascular: Pertaining to the blood vessels of the cerebrum, or brain. [EU]

Cetirizine: A potent second-generation histamine H1 antagonist that is effective in the treatment of allergic rhinitis, chronic urticaria, and pollen-induced asthma. Unlike many traditional antihistamines, it does not cause drowsiness or anticholinergic side effects. [NIH]

Character: In current usage, approximately equivalent to personality. The sum of the relatively fixed personality traits and habitual modes of response of an individual. [NIH]

Chemotherapy: Treatment with anticancer drugs. [NIH]

Chickenpox: A mild, highly contagious virus characterized by itchy blisters all over the body. [NIH]

Chin: The anatomical frontal portion of the mandible, also known as the mentum, that contains the line of fusion of the two separate halves of the mandible (symphysis menti). This line of fusion divides inferiorly to enclose a triangular area called the mental protuberance. On each side, inferior to the second premolar tooth, is the mental foramen for the passage of blood vessels and a nerve. [NIH]

Chlormezanone: A non-benzodiazepine that is used in the management of anxiety. It has been suggested for use in the treatment of muscle spasm. [NIH]

Chlorpheniramine: A histamine H1 antagonist used in allergic reactions, hay fever, rhinitis, urticaria, and asthma. It has also been used in veterinary applications. One of the most widely used of the classical antihistaminics, it generally causes less drowsiness and sedation than promethazine. [NIH]

Chlorpromazine: The prototypical phenothiazine antipsychotic drug. Like the other drugs in this class chlorpromazine's antipsychotic actions are thought to be due to long-term adaptation by the brain to blocking dopamine receptors. Chlorpromazine has several other actions and therapeutic uses, including as an antiemetic and in the treatment of intractable hiccup. [NIH]

Cholangiography: Radiographic examination of the bile ducts. [NIH]

Cholecystography: Radiography of the gallbladder after ingestion of a contrast medium. [NIH]

Cholinergic: Resembling acetylcholine in pharmacological action; stimulated by or releasing acetylcholine or a related compound. [EU]

Cholinergic Agents: Any drug used for its actions on cholinergic systems. Included here are agonists and antagonists, drugs that affect the life cycle of acetylcholine, and drugs that affect the survival of cholinergic neurons. The term cholinergic agents is sometimes still used in the narrower sense of muscarinic agonists, although most modern texts discourage that usage. [NIH]

Chorda Tympani Nerve: A branch of the facial (7th cranial) nerve which passes through the middle ear and continues through the petrotympanic fissure. The chorda tympani nerve carries taste sensation from the anterior two-thirds of the tongue and conveys parasympathetic efferents to the salivary glands. [NIH]

Choroid: The thin, highly vascular membrane covering most of the posterior of the eye between the retina and sclera. [NIH]

Chronic: A disease or condition that persists or progresses over a long period of time. [NIH]

Cimetidine: A histamine congener, it competitively inhibits histamine binding to H2 receptors. Cimetidine has a range of pharmacological actions. It inhibits gastric acid secretion, as well as pepsin and gastrin output. It also blocks the activity of cytochrome P-

450. [NIH]

CIS: Cancer Information Service. The CIS is the National Cancer Institute's link to the public, interpreting and explaining research findings in a clear and understandable manner, and providing personalized responses to specific questions about cancer. Access the CIS by calling 1-800-4-CANCER, or by using the Web site at http://cis.nci.nih.gov. [NIH]

Cisplatin: An inorganic and water-soluble platinum complex. After undergoing hydrolysis, it reacts with DNA to produce both intra and interstrand crosslinks. These crosslinks appear to impair replication and transcription of DNA. The cytotoxicity of cisplatin correlates with cellular arrest in the G2 phase of the cell cycle. [NIH]

Clinical study: A research study in which patients receive treatment in a clinic or other medical facility. Reports of clinical studies can contain results for single patients (case reports) or many patients (case series or clinical trials). [NIH]

Clinical trial: A research study that tests how well new medical treatments or other interventions work in people. Each study is designed to test new methods of screening, prevention, diagnosis, or treatment of a disease. [NIH]

Clonazepam: An anticonvulsant used for several types of seizures, including myotonic or atonic seizures, photosensitive epilepsy, and absence seizures, although tolerance may develop. It is seldom effective in generalized tonic-clonic or partial seizures. The mechanism of action appears to involve the enhancement of gaba receptor responses. [NIH]

Clonic: Pertaining to or of the nature of clonus. [EU]

Cloning: The production of a number of genetically identical individuals; in genetic engineering, a process for the efficient replication of a great number of identical DNA molecules. [NIH]

Coagulation: 1. The process of clot formation. 2. In colloid chemistry, the solidification of a sol into a gelatinous mass; an alteration of a disperse phase or of a dissolved solid which causes the separation of the system into a liquid phase and an insoluble mass called the clot or curd. Coagulation is usually irreversible. 3. In surgery, the disruption of tissue by physical means to form an amorphous residuum, as in electrocoagulation and photocoagulation. [EU]

Coca: Any of several South American shrubs of the Erythroxylon genus (and family) that yield cocaine; the leaves are chewed with alum for CNS stimulation. [NIH]

Cocaine: An alkaloid ester extracted from the leaves of plants including coca. It is a local anesthetic and vasoconstrictor and is clinically used for that purpose, particularly in the eye, ear, nose, and throat. It also has powerful central nervous system effects similar to the amphetamines and is a drug of abuse. Cocaine, like amphetamines, acts by multiple mechanisms on brain catecholaminergic neurons; the mechanism of its reinforcing effects is thought to involve inhibition of dopamine uptake. [NIH]

Cochlea: The part of the internal ear that is concerned with hearing. It forms the anterior part of the labyrinth, is conical, and is placed almost horizontally anterior to the vestibule. [NIH]

Cochlear: Of or pertaining to the cochlea. [EU]

Cochlear Diseases: Diseases of the cochlea, the part of the inner ear that is concerned with hearing. [NIH]

Codeine: An opioid analgesic related to morphine but with less potent analgesic properties and mild sedative effects. It also acts centrally to suppress cough. [NIH]

Cognition: Intellectual or mental process whereby an organism becomes aware of or obtains knowledge. [NIH]

Colic: Paroxysms of pain. This condition usually occurs in the abdominal region but may occur in other body regions as well. [NIH]

Communis: Common tendon of the rectus group of muscles that surrounds the optic foramen and a portion of the superior orbital fissure, to the anterior margin of which it is attached at the spina recti lateralis. [NIH]

Complement: A term originally used to refer to the heat-labile factor in serum that causes immune cytolysis, the lysis of antibody-coated cells, and now referring to the entire functionally related system comprising at least 20 distinct serum proteins that is the effector not only of immune cytolysis but also of other biologic functions. Complement activation occurs by two different sequences, the classic and alternative pathways. The proteins of the classic pathway are termed 'components of complement' and are designated by the symbols C1 through C9. C1 is a calcium-dependent complex of three distinct proteins C1q, C1r and C1s. The proteins of the alternative pathway (collectively referred to as the properdin system) and complement regulatory proteins are known by semisystematic or trivial names. Fragments resulting from proteolytic cleavage of complement proteins are designated with lower-case letter suffixes, e.g., C3a. Inactivated fragments may be designated with the suffix 'i', e.g. C3bi. Activated components or complexes with biological activity are designated by a bar over the symbol e.g. C1 or C4b,2a. The classic pathway is activated by the binding of C1 to classic pathway activators, primarily antigen-antibody complexes containing IgM, IgG1, IgG3; C1q binds to a single IgM molecule or two adjacent IgG molecules. The alternative pathway can be activated by IgA immune complexes and also by nonimmunologic materials including bacterial endotoxins, microbial polysaccharides, and cell walls. Activation of the classic pathway triggers an enzymatic cascade involving C1, C4, C2 and C3; activation of the alternative pathway triggers a cascade involving C3 and factors B, D and P. Both result in the cleavage of C5 and the formation of the membrane attack complex. Complement activation also results in the formation of many biologically active complement fragments that act as anaphylatoxins, opsonins, or chemotactic factors. [EU]

Complementary and alternative medicine: CAM. Forms of treatment that are used in addition to (complementary) or instead of (alternative) standard treatments. These practices are not considered standard medical approaches. CAM includes dietary supplements, megadose vitamins, herbal preparations, special teas, massage therapy, magnet therapy, spiritual healing, and meditation. [NIH]

Complementary medicine: Practices not generally recognized by the medical community as standard or conventional medical approaches and used to enhance or complement the standard treatments. Complementary medicine includes the taking of dietary supplements, megadose vitamins, and herbal preparations; the drinking of special teas; and practices such as massage therapy, magnet therapy, spiritual healing, and meditation. [NIH]

Complete remission: The disappearance of all signs of cancer. Also called a complete response. [NIH]

Computational Biology: A field of biology concerned with the development of techniques for the collection and manipulation of biological data, and the use of such data to make biological discoveries or predictions. This field encompasses all computational methods and theories applicable to molecular biology and areas of computer-based techniques for solving biological problems including manipulation of models and datasets. [NIH]

Conception: The onset of pregnancy, marked by implantation of the blastocyst; the formation of a viable zygote. [EU]

Confusion: A mental state characterized by bewilderment, emotional disturbance, lack of clear thinking, and perceptual disorientation. [NIH]

Congestion: Excessive or abnormal accumulation of blood in a part. [EU]

Conjugated: Acting or operating as if joined; simultaneous. [EU]

Conjunctiva: The mucous membrane that lines the inner surface of the eyelids and the anterior part of the sclera. [NIH]

Conjunctivitis: Inflammation of the conjunctiva, generally consisting of conjunctival hyperaemia associated with a discharge. [EU]

Consciousness: Sense of awareness of self and of the environment. [NIH]

Constipation: Infrequent or difficult evacuation of feces. [NIH]

Contact dermatitis: Inflammation of the skin with varying degrees of erythema, edema and vesinculation resulting from cutaneous contact with a foreign substance or other exposure. [NIH]

Contraindications: Any factor or sign that it is unwise to pursue a certain kind of action or treatment, e. g. giving a general anesthetic to a person with pneumonia. [NIH]

Contrast Media: Substances used in radiography that allow visualization of certain tissues. [NIH]

Contrast medium: A substance that is introduced into or around a structure and, because of the difference in absorption of x-rays by the contrast medium and the surrounding tissues, allows radiographic visualization of the structure. [EU]

Coordination: Muscular or motor regulation or the harmonious cooperation of muscles or groups of muscles, in a complex action or series of actions. [NIH]

Cornea: The transparent part of the eye that covers the iris and the pupil and allows light to enter the inside. [NIH]

Cortex: The outer layer of an organ or other body structure, as distinguished from the internal substance. [EU]

Cortical: Pertaining to or of the nature of a cortex or bark. [EU]

Cortisone: A natural steroid hormone produced in the adrenal gland. It can also be made in the laboratory. Cortisone reduces swelling and can suppress immune responses. [NIH]

Cranial: Pertaining to the cranium, or to the anterior (in animals) or superior (in humans) end of the body. [EU]

Craniocerebral Trauma: Traumatic injuries involving the cranium and intracranial structures (i.e., brain; cranial nerves; meninges; and other structures). Injuries may be classified by whether or not the skull is penetrated (i.e., penetrating vs. nonpenetrating) or whether there is an associated hemorrhage. [NIH]

Curative: Tending to overcome disease and promote recovery. [EU]

Cutaneous: Having to do with the skin. [NIH]

Cyanide: An extremely toxic class of compounds that can be lethal on inhaling of ingesting in minute quantities. [NIH]

Cyclic: Pertaining to or occurring in a cycle or cycles; the term is applied to chemical compounds that contain a ring of atoms in the nucleus. [EU]

Cyclophosphamide: Precursor of an alkylating nitrogen mustard antineoplastic and immunosuppressive agent that must be activated in the liver to form the active aldophosphamide. It is used in the treatment of lymphomas, leukemias, etc. Its side effect, alopecia, has been made use of in defleecing sheep. Cyclophosphamide may also cause sterility, birth defects, mutations, and cancer. [NIH]

Cytochrome: Any electron transfer hemoprotein having a mode of action in which the transfer of a single electron is effected by a reversible valence change of the central iron atom of the heme prosthetic group between the +2 and +3 oxidation states; classified as cytochromes a in which the heme contains a formyl side chain, cytochromes b, which contain protoheme or a closely similar heme that is not covalently bound to the protein, cytochromes c in which protoheme or other heme is covalently bound to the protein, and cytochromes d in which the iron-tetrapyrrole has fewer conjugated double bonds than the hemes have. Well-known cytochromes have been numbered consecutively within groups and are designated by subscripts (beginning with no subscript), e.g. cytochromes c, c1, C2, . New cytochromes are named according to the wavelength in nanometres of the absorption maximum of the a-band of the iron (II) form in pyridine, e.g., c-555. [EU]

Cytoplasm: The protoplasm of a cell exclusive of that of the nucleus; it consists of a continuous aqueous solution (cytosol) and the organelles and inclusions suspended in it (phaneroplasm), and is the site of most of the chemical activities of the cell. [EU]

Cytotoxic: Cell-killing. [NIH]

Cytotoxic chemotherapy: Anticancer drugs that kill cells, especially cancer cells. [NIH]

Cytotoxicity: Quality of being capable of producing a specific toxic action upon cells of special organs. [NIH]

Decarboxylation: The removal of a carboxyl group, usually in the form of carbon dioxide, from a chemical compound. [NIH]

Decongestant: An agent that reduces congestion or swelling. [EU]

Degenerative: Undergoing degeneration : tending to degenerate; having the character of or involving degeneration; causing or tending to cause degeneration. [EU]

Delirium: (DSM III-R) an acute, reversible organic mental disorder characterized by reduced ability to maintain attention to external stimuli and disorganized thinking as manifested by rambling, irrelevant, or incoherent speech; there are also a reduced level of consciousness, sensory misperceptions, disturbance of the sleep-wakefulness cycle and level of psychomotor activity, disorientation to time, place, or person, and memory impairment. Delirium may be caused by a large number of conditions resulting in derangement of cerebral metabolism, including systemic infection, poisoning, drug intoxication or withdrawal, seizures or head trauma, and metabolic disturbances such as hypoxia, hypoglycaemia, fluid, electrolyte, or acid-base imbalances, or hepatic or renal failure. Called also acute confusional state and acute brain syndrome. [EU]

Delusions: A false belief regarding the self or persons or objects outside the self that persists despite the facts, and is not considered tenable by one's associates. [NIH]

Dementia: An acquired organic mental disorder with loss of intellectual abilities of sufficient severity to interfere with social or occupational functioning. The dysfunction is multifaceted and involves memory, behavior, personality, judgment, attention, spatial relations, language, abstract thought, and other executive functions. The intellectual decline is usually progressive, and initially spares the level of consciousness. [NIH]

Dendrites: Extensions of the nerve cell body. They are short and branched and receive stimuli from other neurons. [NIH]

Dermatitis: Any inflammation of the skin. [NIH]

Dermatosis: Any skin disease, especially one not characterized by inflammation. [EU]

Dermis: A layer of vascular connective tissue underneath the epidermis. The surface of the dermis contains sensitive papillae. Embedded in or beneath the dermis are sweat glands, hair follicles, and sebaceous glands. [NIH]

Detoxification: Treatment designed to free an addict from his drug habit. [EU]

Deuterium: Deuterium. The stable isotope of hydrogen. It has one neutron and one proton in the nucleus. [NIH]

Dexamethasone: (11 beta,16 alpha)-9-Fluoro-11,17,21-trihydroxy-16-methylpregna-1,4-diene-3,20-dione. An anti-inflammatory glucocorticoid used either in the free alcohol or esterified form in treatment of conditions that respond generally to cortisone. [NIH]

Dextroamphetamine: The d-form of amphetamine. It is a central nervous system stimulant and a sympathomimetic. It has also been used in the treatment of narcolepsy and of attention deficit disorders and hyperactivity in children. Dextroamphetamine has multiple mechanisms of action including blocking uptake of adrenergics and dopamine, stimulating release of monamines, and inhibiting monoamine oxidase. It is also a drug of abuse and a psychotomimetic. [NIH]

Dextromethorphan: The d-isomer of the codeine analog of levorphanol. Dextromethorphan shows high affinity binding to several regions of the brain, including the medullary cough center. This compound is a NMDA receptor antagonist (receptors, N-methyl-D-aspartate) and acts as a non-competitive channel blocker. It is used widely as an antitussive agent, and is also used to study the involvement of glutamate receptors in neurotoxicity. [NIH]

Diagnostic procedure: A method used to identify a disease. [NIH]

Dialyzer: A part of the hemodialysis machine. (See hemodialysis under dialysis.) The dialyzer has two sections separated by a membrane. One section holds dialysate. The other holds the patient's blood. [NIH]

Diastolic: Of or pertaining to the diastole. [EU]

Diethylcarbamazine: An anthelmintic used primarily as the citrate in the treatment of filariasis, particularly infestations with Wucheria bancrofti or Loa loa. [NIH]

Diflunisal: A salicylate derivative and anti-inflammatory analgesic with actions and side effects similar to those of aspirin. [NIH]

Digestion: The process of breakdown of food for metabolism and use by the body. [NIH]

Digestive system: The organs that take in food and turn it into products that the body can use to stay healthy. Waste products the body cannot use leave the body through bowel movements. The digestive system includes the salivary glands, mouth, esophagus, stomach, liver, pancreas, gallbladder, small and large intestines, and rectum. [NIH]

Digestive tract: The organs through which food passes when food is eaten. These organs are the mouth, esophagus, stomach, small and large intestines, and rectum. [NIH]

Dimenhydrinate: A drug combination that contains diphenhydramine and theophylline. It is used for treating vertigo, motion sickness, and nausea associated with pregnancy. It is not effective in the treatment of nausea associated with cancer chemotherapy. [NIH]

Diploid: Having two sets of chromosomes. [NIH]

Direct: 1. Straight; in a straight line. 2. Performed immediately and without the intervention of subsidiary means. [EU]

Discrete: Made up of separate parts or characterized by lesions which do not become blended; not running together; separate. [NIH]

Disinfectant: An agent that disinfects; applied particularly to agents used on inanimate objects. [EU]

Disorientation: The loss of proper bearings, or a state of mental confusion as to time, place, or identity. [EU]

Disposition: A tendency either physical or mental toward certain diseases. [EU]

Dissociation: 1. The act of separating or state of being separated. 2. The separation of a molecule into two or more fragments (atoms, molecules, ions, or free radicals) produced by the absorption of light or thermal energy or by solvation. 3. In psychology, a defense mechanism in which a group of mental processes are segregated from the rest of a person's mental activity in order to avoid emotional distress, as in the dissociative disorders (q.v.), or in which an idea or object is segregated from its emotional significance; in the first sense it is roughly equivalent to splitting, in the second, to isolation. 4. A defect of mental integration in which one or more groups of mental processes become separated off from normal consciousness and, thus separated, function as a unitary whole. [EU]

Diuresis: Increased excretion of urine. [EU]

Dizziness: An imprecise term which may refer to a sense of spatial disorientation, motion of the environment, or lightheadedness. [NIH]

Dopamine: An endogenous catecholamine and prominent neurotransmitter in several systems of the brain. In the synthesis of catecholamines from tyrosine, it is the immediate precursor to norepinephrine and epinephrine. Dopamine is a major transmitter in the extrapyramidal system of the brain, and important in regulating movement. A family of dopaminergic receptor subtypes mediate its action. Dopamine is used pharmacologically for its direct (beta adrenergic agonist) and indirect (adrenergic releasing) sympathomimetic effects including its actions as an inotropic agent and as a renal vasodilator. [NIH]

Dosage Forms: Completed forms of the pharmaceutical preparation in which prescribed doses of medication are included. They are designed to resist action by gastric fluids, prevent vomiting and nausea, reduce or alleviate the undesirable taste and smells associated with oral administration, achieve a high concentration of drug at target site, or produce a delayed or long-acting drug effect. They include capsules, liniments, ointments, pharmaceutical solutions, powders, tablets, etc. [NIH]

Double-blind: Pertaining to a clinical trial or other experiment in which neither the subject nor the person administering treatment knows which treatment any particular subject is receiving. [EU]

Doxepin: A dibenzoxepin tricyclic compound. It displays a range of pharmacological actions including maintaining adrenergic innervation. Its mechanism of action is not fully understood, but it appears to block reuptake of monoaminergic neurotransmitters into presynaptic terminals. It also possesses anticholinergic activity and modulates antagonism of histamine H(1)- and H(2)-receptors. [NIH]

Drive: A state of internal activity of an organism that is a necessary condition before a given stimulus will elicit a class of responses; e.g., a certain level of hunger (drive) must be present before food will elicit an eating response. [NIH]

Dross: Residue remaining in an opium pipe which has been smoked; contains 50 % of the morphine present in the original drug. [NIH]

Drug Interactions: The action of a drug that may affect the activity, metabolism, or toxicity of another drug. [NIH]

Drug Tolerance: Progressive diminution of the susceptibility of a human or animal to the effects of a drug, resulting from its continued administration. It should be differentiated from drug resistance wherein an organism, disease, or tissue fails to respond to the intended effectiveness of a chemical or drug. It should also be differentiated from maximum tolerated dose and no-observed-adverse-effect level. [NIH]

Duct: A tube through which body fluids pass. [NIH]

Duodenal Ulcer: An ulcer in the lining of the first part of the small intestine (duodenum). [NIH]

Duodenum: The first part of the small intestine. [NIH]

Dyskinesia: Impairment of the power of voluntary movement, resulting in fragmentary or incomplete movements. [EU]

Dysmenorrhea: Painful menstruation. [NIH]

Dyspepsia: Impaired digestion, especially after eating. [NIH]

Dystonia: Disordered tonicity of muscle. [EU]

Eccrine Glands: Simple sweat glands that secrete sweat directly onto the skin. [NIH]

Edema: Excessive amount of watery fluid accumulated in the intercellular spaces, most commonly present in subcutaneous tissue. [NIH]

Effector: It is often an enzyme that converts an inactive precursor molecule into an active second messenger. [NIH]

Effector cell: A cell that performs a specific function in response to a stimulus; usually used to describe cells in the immune system. [NIH]

Efficacy: The extent to which a specific intervention, procedure, regimen, or service produces a beneficial result under ideal conditions. Ideally, the determination of efficacy is based on the results of a randomized control trial. [NIH]

Elastic: Susceptible of resisting and recovering from stretching, compression or distortion applied by a force. [EU]

Electrocoagulation: Electrosurgical procedures used to treat hemorrhage (e.g., bleeding ulcers) and to ablate tumors, mucosal lesions, and refractory arrhythmias. [NIH]

Electrolyte: A substance that dissociates into ions when fused or in solution, and thus becomes capable of conducting electricity; an ionic solute. [EU]

Electrons: Stable elementary particles having the smallest known negative charge, present in all elements; also called negatrons. Positively charged electrons are called positrons. The numbers, energies and arrangement of electrons around atomic nuclei determine the chemical identities of elements. Beams of electrons are called cathode rays or beta rays, the latter being a high-energy biproduct of nuclear decay. [NIH]

Emesis: Vomiting; an act of vomiting. Also used as a word termination, as in haematemesis. [EU]

Emodin: Purgative anthraquinone found in several plants, especially Rhamnus frangula. It was formerly used as a laxative, but is now used mainly as tool in toxicity studies. [NIH]

Emollient: Softening or soothing; called also malactic. [EU]

Encapsulated: Confined to a specific, localized area and surrounded by a thin layer of tissue. [NIH]

Encephalitis: Inflammation of the brain due to infection, autoimmune processes, toxins, and other conditions. Viral infections (see encephalitis, viral) are a relatively frequent cause of this condition. [NIH]

Encephalitis, Viral: Inflammation of brain parenchymal tissue as a result of viral infection. Encephalitis may occur as primary or secondary manifestation of Togaviridae infections; Herpesviridae infections; Adenoviridae infections; Flaviviridae infections; Bunyaviridae infections; Picornaviridae infections; Paramyxoviridae infections; Orthomyxoviridae infections; Retroviridae infections; and Arenaviridae infections. [NIH]

Encephalopathy: A disorder of the brain that can be caused by disease, injury, drugs, or chemicals. [NIH]

Endogenous: Produced inside an organism or cell. The opposite is external (exogenous) production. [NIH]

Enhancer: Transcriptional element in the virus genome. [NIH]

Enterohepatic: Of or involving the intestine and liver. [EU]

Enterohepatic Circulation: Recycling through liver by excretion in bile, reabsorption from intestines into portal circulation, passage back into liver, and re-excretion in bile. [NIH]

Environmental Health: The science of controlling or modifying those conditions, influences, or forces surrounding man which relate to promoting, establishing, and maintaining health. [NIH]

Enzymatic: Phase where enzyme cuts the precursor protein. [NIH]

Enzyme: A protein that speeds up chemical reactions in the body. [NIH]

Epidermis: Nonvascular layer of the skin. It is made up, from within outward, of five layers: 1) basal layer (stratum basale epidermidis); 2) spinous layer (stratum spinosum epidermidis); 3) granular layer (stratum granulosum epidermidis); 4) clear layer (stratum lucidum epidermidis); and 5) horny layer (stratum corneum epidermidis). [NIH]

Epinephrine: The active sympathomimetic hormone from the adrenal medulla in most species. It stimulates both the alpha- and beta- adrenergic systems, causes systemic vasoconstriction and gastrointestinal relaxation, stimulates the heart, and dilates bronchi and cerebral vessels. It is used in asthma and cardiac failure and to delay absorption of local anesthetics. [NIH]

Epithelial: Refers to the cells that line the internal and external surfaces of the body. [NIH]

Epithelium: One or more layers of epithelial cells, supported by the basal lamina, which covers the inner or outer surfaces of the body. [NIH]

Erythema: Redness of the skin produced by congestion of the capillaries. This condition may result from a variety of causes. [NIH]

Erythrocytes: Red blood cells. Mature erythrocytes are non-nucleated, biconcave disks containing hemoglobin whose function is to transport oxygen. [NIH]

Esophagitis: Inflammation, acute or chronic, of the esophagus caused by bacteria, chemicals, or trauma. [NIH]

Esophagus: The muscular tube through which food passes from the throat to the stomach. [NIH]

Estrogen: One of the two female sex hormones. [NIH]

Ethanol: A clear, colorless liquid rapidly absorbed from the gastrointestinal tract and distributed throughout the body. It has bactericidal activity and is used often as a topical disinfectant. It is widely used as a solvent and preservative in pharmaceutical preparations as well as serving as the primary ingredient in alcoholic beverages. [NIH]

Ethanolamine: A viscous, hygroscopic amino alcohol with an ammoniacal odor. It is widely distributed in biological tissue and is a component of lecithin. It is used as a surfactant, fluorimetric reagent, and to remove CO_2 and H_2S from natural gas and other gases. [NIH]

Ether: One of a class of organic compounds in which any two organic radicals are attached directly to a single oxygen atom. [NIH]

Excipients: Usually inert substances added to a prescription in order to provide suitable consistency to the dosage form; a binder, matrix, base or diluent in pills, tablets, creams, salves, etc. [NIH]

Excitability: Property of a cardiac cell whereby, when the cell is depolarized to a critical level (called threshold), the membrane becomes permeable and a regenerative inward current causes an action potential. [NIH]

Excitation: An act of irritation or stimulation or of responding to a stimulus; the addition of energy, as the excitation of a molecule by absorption of photons. [EU]

Excitatory: When cortical neurons are excited, their output increases and each new input they receive while they are still excited raises their output markedly. [NIH]

Exhaustion: The feeling of weariness of mind and body. [NIH]

Exogenous: Developed or originating outside the organism, as exogenous disease. [EU]

Extracellular: Outside a cell or cells. [EU]

Extracorporeal: Situated or occurring outside the body. [EU]

Extrapyramidal: Outside of the pyramidal tracts. [EU]

Eye Movements: Voluntary or reflex-controlled movements of the eye. [NIH]

Facial: Of or pertaining to the face. [EU]

Facial Nerve: The 7th cranial nerve. The facial nerve has two parts, the larger motor root which may be called the facial nerve proper, and the smaller intermediate or sensory root. Together they provide efferent innervation to the muscles of facial expression and to the lacrimal and salivary glands, and convey afferent information for taste from the anterior two-thirds of the tongue and for touch from the external ear. [NIH]

Family Planning: Programs or services designed to assist the family in controlling reproduction by either improving or diminishing fertility. [NIH]

Family Practice: A medical specialty concerned with the provision of continuing, comprehensive primary health care for the entire family. [NIH]

Famotidine: A competitive histamine H2-receptor antagonist. Its main pharmacodynamic effect is the inhibition of gastric secretion. [NIH]

Fat: Total lipids including phospholipids. [NIH]

Fatigue: The state of weariness following a period of exertion, mental or physical, characterized by a decreased capacity for work and reduced efficiency to respond to stimuli. [NIH]

Fenoprofen: An anti-inflammatory analgesic and antipyretic highly bound to plasma proteins. It is pharmacologically similar to aspirin, but causes less gastrointestinal bleeding. [NIH]

Fetus: The developing offspring from 7 to 8 weeks after conception until birth. [NIH]

Fibrin: A protein derived from fibrinogen in the presence of thrombin, which forms part of the blood clot. [NIH]

Fibrosis: Any pathological condition where fibrous connective tissue invades any organ, usually as a consequence of inflammation or other injury. [NIH]

Filariasis: Infections with nematodes of the superfamily Filarioidea. The presence of living worms in the body is mainly asymptomatic but the death of adult worms leads to granulomatous inflammation and permanent fibrosis. Organisms of the genus Elaeophora infect wild elk and domestic sheep causing ischaemic necrosis of the brain, blindness, and dermatosis of the face. [NIH]

Fixation: 1. The act or operation of holding, suturing, or fastening in a fixed position. 2. The condition of being held in a fixed position. 3. In psychiatry, a term with two related but distinct meanings : (1) arrest of development at a particular stage, which like regression (return to an earlier stage), if temporary is a normal reaction to setbacks and difficulties but if protracted or frequent is a cause of developmental failures and emotional problems, and (2) a close and suffocating attachment to another person, especially a childhood figure, such as one's mother or father. Both meanings are derived from psychoanalytic theory and refer to 'fixation' of libidinal energy either in a specific erogenous zone, hence fixation at the oral, anal, or phallic stage, or in a specific object, hence mother or father fixation. 4. The use of a fixative (q.v.) to preserve histological or cytological specimens. 5. In chemistry, the process whereby a substance is removed from the gaseous or solution phase and localized, as in carbon dioxide fixation or nitrogen fixation. 6. In ophthalmology, direction of the gaze so that the visual image of the object falls on the fovea centralis. 7. In film processing, the chemical removal of all undeveloped salts of the film emulsion, leaving only the developed silver to form a permanent image. [EU]

Flatus: Gas passed through the rectum. [NIH]

Fluorescence: The property of emitting radiation while being irradiated. The radiation emitted is usually of longer wavelength than that incident or absorbed, e.g., a substance can be irradiated with invisible radiation and emit visible light. X-ray fluorescence is used in diagnosis. [NIH]

Fluoxetine: The first highly specific serotonin uptake inhibitor. It is used as an antidepressant and often has a more acceptable side-effects profile than traditional antidepressants. [NIH]

Fluphenazine: A phenothiazine used in the treatment of psychoses. Its properties and uses are generally similar to those of chlorpromazine. [NIH]

Flurazepam: A benzodiazepine derivative used mainly as a hypnotic. [NIH]

Flurbiprofen: An anti-inflammatory analgesic and antipyretic of the phenylalkynoic acid series. It has been shown to reduce bone resorption in periodontal disease by inhibiting carbonic anhydrase. [NIH]

GABA: The most common inhibitory neurotransmitter in the central nervous system. [NIH]

Gamma Rays: Very powerful and penetrating, high-energy electromagnetic radiation of shorter wavelength than that of x-rays. They are emitted by a decaying nucleus, usually between 0.01 and 10 MeV. They are also called nuclear x-rays. [NIH]

Ganglia: Clusters of multipolar neurons surrounded by a capsule of loosely organized connective tissue located outside the central nervous system. [NIH]

Ganglion: 1. A knot, or knotlike mass. 2. A general term for a group of nerve cell bodies located outside the central nervous system; occasionally applied to certain nuclear groups within the brain or spinal cord, e.g. basal ganglia. 3. A benign cystic tumour occurring on a aponeurosis or tendon, as in the wrist or dorsum of the foot; it consists of a thin fibrous capsule enclosing a clear mucinous fluid. [EU]

Gas: Air that comes from normal breakdown of food. The gases are passed out of the body through the rectum (flatus) or the mouth (burp). [NIH]

Gas exchange: Primary function of the lungs; transfer of oxygen from inhaled air into the blood and of carbon dioxide from the blood into the lungs. [NIH]

Gastric: Having to do with the stomach. [NIH]

Gastric Acid: Hydrochloric acid present in gastric juice. [NIH]

Gastrin: A hormone released after eating. Gastrin causes the stomach to produce more acid. [NIH]

Gastritis: Inflammation of the stomach. [EU]

Gastrointestinal: Refers to the stomach and intestines. [NIH]

Gastrointestinal tract: The stomach and intestines. [NIH]

Gene: The functional and physical unit of heredity passed from parent to offspring. Genes are pieces of DNA, and most genes contain the information for making a specific protein. [NIH]

Genital: Pertaining to the genitalia. [EU]

Gentian Violet: A dye that is a mixture of violet rosanilinis with antibacterial, antifungal, and anthelmentic properties. [NIH]

Gestation: The period of development of the young in viviparous animals, from the time of fertilization of the ovum until birth. [EU]

Gland: An organ that produces and releases one or more substances for use in the body. Some glands produce fluids that affect tissues or organs. Others produce hormones or participate in blood production. [NIH]

Glossopharyngeal Nerve: The 9th cranial nerve. The glossopharyngeal nerve is a mixed motor and sensory nerve; it conveys somatic and autonomic efferents as well as general, special, and visceral afferents. Among the connections are motor fibers to the stylopharyngeus muscle, parasympathetic fibers to the parotid glands, general and taste afferents from the posterior third of the tongue, the nasopharynx, and the palate, and afferents from baroreceptors and chemoreceptors of the carotid sinus. [NIH]

Glottis: The vocal apparatus of the larynx, consisting of the true vocal cords (plica vocalis) and the opening between them (rima glottidis). [NIH]

Glucocorticoid: A compound that belongs to the family of compounds called corticosteroids (steroids). Glucocorticoids affect metabolism and have anti-inflammatory and immunosuppressive effects. They may be naturally produced (hormones) or synthetic (drugs). [NIH]

Glucuronic Acid: Derivatives of uronic acid found throughout the plant and animal kingdoms. They detoxify drugs and toxins by conjugating with them to form glucuronides in the liver which are more water-soluble metabolites that can be easily eliminated from the body. [NIH]

Glucuronides: Glycosides of glucuronic acid formed by the reaction of uridine diphosphate glucuronic acid with certain endogenous and exogenous substances. Their formation is important for the detoxification of drugs, steroid excretion and bilirubin metabolism to a more water-soluble compound that can be eliminated in the urine and bile. [NIH]

Glutamate: Excitatory neurotransmitter of the brain. [NIH]

Glutamic Acid: A non-essential amino acid naturally occurring in the L-form. Glutamic acid (glutamate) is the most common excitatory neurotransmitter in the central nervous system. [NIH]

Glycerol: A trihydroxy sugar alcohol that is an intermediate in carbohydrate and lipid metabolism. It is used as a solvent, emollient, pharmaceutical agent, and sweetening agent. [NIH]

Glycols: A generic grouping for dihydric alcohols with the hydroxy groups (-OH) located on different carbon atoms. They are viscous liquids with high boiling points for their molecular weights. [NIH]

Glycopyrrolate: A muscarinic antagonist used as an antispasmodic, in some disorders of the gastrointestinal tract, and to reduce salivation with some anesthetics. [NIH]

Gout: Hereditary metabolic disorder characterized by recurrent acute arthritis, hyperuricemia and deposition of sodium urate in and around the joints, sometimes with formation of uric acid calculi. [NIH]

Governing Board: The group in which legal authority is vested for the control of health-related institutions and organizations. [NIH]

Gram-negative: Losing the stain or decolorized by alcohol in Gram's method of staining, a primary characteristic of bacteria having a cell wall composed of a thin layer of peptidoglycan covered by an outer membrane of lipoprotein and lipopolysaccharide. [EU]

Gram-positive: Retaining the stain or resisting decolorization by alcohol in Gram's method of staining, a primary characteristic of bacteria whose cell wall is composed of a thick layer of peptidologlycan with attached teichoic acids. [EU]

Granisetron: A serotonin receptor (5HT-3 selective) antagonist that has been used as an antiemetic for cancer chemotherapy patients. [NIH]

Habitual: Of the nature of a habit; according to habit; established by or repeated by force of habit, customary. [EU]

Haematemesis: The vomiting of blood. [EU]

Haemoperfusion: 1. The act of pouring over or through, especially the passage of blood through the vessels of a specific organ. 2. Blood poured over or through an organ or tissue. [EU]

Hair follicles: Shafts or openings on the surface of the skin through which hair grows. [NIH]

Half-Life: The time it takes for a substance (drug, radioactive nuclide, or other) to lose half of its pharmacologic, physiologic, or radiologic activity. [NIH]

Hallucinogen: A hallucination-producing drug, a category of drugs producing this effect. The user of a hallucinogenic drug is almost invariably aware that what he is seeing are hallucinations. [NIH]

Haloperidol: Butyrophenone derivative. [NIH]

Haploid: An organism with one basic chromosome set, symbolized by n; the normal condition of gametes in diploids. [NIH]

Haptens: Small antigenic determinants capable of eliciting an immune response only when coupled to a carrier. Haptens bind to antibodies but by themselves cannot elicit an antibody response. [NIH]

Hay Fever: A seasonal variety of allergic rhinitis, marked by acute conjunctivitis with lacrimation and itching, regarded as an allergic condition triggered by specific allergens. [NIH]

Headache: Pain in the cranial region that may occur as an isolated and benign symptom or as a manifestation of a wide variety of conditions including subarachnoid hemorrhage; craniocerebral trauma; central nervous system infections; intracranial hypertension; and other disorders. In general, recurrent headaches that are not associated with a primary disease process are referred to as headache disorders (e.g., migraine). [NIH]

Headache Disorders: Common conditions characterized by persistent or recurrent headaches. Headache syndrome classification systems may be based on etiology (e.g., vascular headache, post-traumatic headaches, etc.), temporal pattern (e.g., cluster headache, paroxysmal hemicrania, etc.), and precipitating factors (e.g., cough headache). [NIH]

Heartburn: Substernal pain or burning sensation, usually associated with regurgitation of gastric juice into the esophagus. [NIH]

Hemodialysis: The use of a machine to clean wastes from the blood after the kidneys have failed. The blood travels through tubes to a dialyzer, which removes wastes and extra fluid. The cleaned blood then flows through another set of tubes back into the body. [NIH]

Hemoperfusion: Removal of toxins or metabolites from the circulation by the passing of blood, within a suitable extracorporeal circuit, over semipermeable microcapsules containing adsorbents (e.g., activated charcoal) or enzymes, other enzyme preparations (e.g., gel-entrapped microsomes, membrane-free enzymes bound to artificial carriers), or other adsorbents (e.g., various resins, albumin-conjugated agarose). [NIH]

Hemophilia: Refers to a group of hereditary disorders in which affected individuals fail to make enough of certain proteins needed to form blood clots. [NIH]

Hemorrhage: Bleeding or escape of blood from a vessel. [NIH]

Hemostasis: The process which spontaneously arrests the flow of blood from vessels carrying blood under pressure. It is accomplished by contraction of the vessels, adhesion and aggregation of formed blood elements, and the process of blood or plasma coagulation. [NIH]

Hepatic: Refers to the liver. [NIH]

Hereditary: Of, relating to, or denoting factors that can be transmitted genetically from one generation to another. [NIH]

Herpes: Any inflammatory skin disease caused by a herpesvirus and characterized by the formation of clusters of small vesicles. When used alone, the term may refer to herpes simplex or to herpes zoster. [EU]

Herpes Zoster: Acute vesicular inflammation. [NIH]

Heterogeneity: The property of one or more samples or populations which implies that they are not identical in respect of some or all of their parameters, e. g. heterogeneity of variance. [NIH]

Hirsutism: Excess hair in females and children with an adult male pattern of distribution. The concept does not include hypertrichosis, which is localized or generalized excess hair. [NIH]

Histamine: 1H-Imidazole-4-ethanamine. A depressor amine derived by enzymatic decarboxylation of histidine. It is a powerful stimulant of gastric secretion, a constrictor of bronchial smooth muscle, a vasodilator, and also a centrally acting neurotransmitter. [NIH]

Histidine: An essential amino acid important in a number of metabolic processes. It is required for the production of histamine. [NIH]

Homogeneous: Consisting of or composed of similar elements or ingredients; of a uniform quality throughout. [EU]

Homologous: Corresponding in structure, position, origin, etc., as (a) the feathers of a bird and the scales of a fish, (b) antigen and its specific antibody, (c) allelic chromosomes. [EU]

Hormone: A substance in the body that regulates certain organs. Hormones such as gastrin help in breaking down food. Some hormones come from cells in the stomach and small intestine. [NIH]

Hydrofluoric Acid: A solution of hydrogen fluoride in water. It is a colorless fuming liquid which can cause painful burns. [NIH]

Hydrogen: The first chemical element in the periodic table. It has the atomic symbol H, atomic number 1, and atomic weight 1. It exists, under normal conditions, as a colorless, odorless, tasteless, diatomic gas. Hydrogen ions are protons. Besides the common H1 isotope, hydrogen exists as the stable isotope deuterium and the unstable, radioactive isotope tritium. [NIH]

Hydrogen Peroxide: A strong oxidizing agent used in aqueous solution as a ripening agent, bleach, and topical anti-infective. It is relatively unstable and solutions deteriorate over time unless stabilized by the addition of acetanilide or similar organic materials. [NIH]

Hydrogenation: Specific method of reduction in which hydrogen is added to a substance by the direct use of gaseous hydrogen. [NIH]

Hydrolysis: The process of cleaving a chemical compound by the addition of a molecule of water. [NIH]

Hydrophilic: Readily absorbing moisture; hygroscopic; having strongly polar groups that readily interact with water. [EU]

Hyperaemia: An excess of blood in a part; engorgement. [EU]

Hyperemesis: Excessive vomiting. [EU]

Hypersensitivity: Altered reactivity to an antigen, which can result in pathologic reactions upon subsequent exposure to that particular antigen. [NIH]

Hypertension: Persistently high arterial blood pressure. Currently accepted threshold levels are 140 mm Hg systolic and 90 mm Hg diastolic pressure. [NIH]

Hypertrichosis: Localized or generalized excess hair. The concept does not include hirsutism, which is excess hair in females and children with an adult male pattern of distribution. [NIH]

Hypnotic: A drug that acts to induce sleep. [EU]

Hypodermic: Applied or administered beneath the skin. [EU]

Hypoglycaemia: An abnormally diminished concentration of glucose in the blood, which may lead to tremulousness, cold sweat, piloerection, hypothermia, and headache, accompanied by irritability, confusion, hallucinations, bizarre behaviour, and ultimately, convulsions and coma. [EU]

Hypotension: Abnormally low blood pressure. [NIH]

Hypoxia: Reduction of oxygen supply to tissue below physiological levels despite adequate perfusion of the tissue by blood. [EU]

Hypoxic: Having too little oxygen. [NIH]

Ibuprofen: A nonsteroidal anti-inflammatory agent with analgesic properties used in the therapy of rheumatism and arthritis. [NIH]

Idiopathic: Describes a disease of unknown cause. [NIH]

Illusion: A false interpretation of a genuine percept. [NIH]

Imidazole: C3H4N2. The ring is present in polybenzimidazoles. [NIH]

Immune response: The activity of the immune system against foreign substances (antigens). [NIH]

Immune system: The organs, cells, and molecules responsible for the recognition and disposal of foreign ("non-self") material which enters the body. [NIH]

Immunization: Deliberate stimulation of the host's immune response. Active immunization involves administration of antigens or immunologic adjuvants. Passive immunization involves administration of immune sera or lymphocytes or their extracts (e.g., transfer factor, immune RNA) or transplantation of immunocompetent cell producing tissue (thymus or bone marrow). [NIH]

Immunoassay: Immunochemical assay or detection of a substance by serologic or immunologic methods. Usually the substance being studied serves as antigen both in antibody production and in measurement of antibody by the test substance. [NIH]

Immunologic: The ability of the antibody-forming system to recall a previous experience with an antigen and to respond to a second exposure with the prompt production of large amounts of antibody. [NIH]

Immunology: The study of the body's immune system. [NIH]

Immunosuppressant: An agent capable of suppressing immune responses. [EU]

Immunosuppressive: Describes the ability to lower immune system responses. [NIH]

Impairment: In the context of health experience, an impairment is any loss or abnormality of psychological, physiological, or anatomical structure or function. [NIH]

In vivo: In the body. The opposite of in vitro (outside the body or in the laboratory). [NIH]

Incontinence: Inability to control the flow of urine from the bladder (urinary incontinence) or the escape of stool from the rectum (fecal incontinence). [NIH]

Incubation: The development of an infectious disease from the entrance of the pathogen to the appearance of clinical symptoms. [EU]

Incubation period: The period of time likely to elapse between exposure to the agent of the disease and the onset of clinical symptoms. [NIH]

Indigestion: Poor digestion. Symptoms include heartburn, nausea, bloating, and gas. Also called dyspepsia. [NIH]

Infancy: The period of complete dependency prior to the acquisition of competence in walking, talking, and self-feeding. [NIH]

Infection: 1. Invasion and multiplication of microorganisms in body tissues, which may be clinically unapparent or result in local cellular injury due to competitive metabolism, toxins, intracellular replication, or antigen-antibody response. The infection may remain localized, subclinical, and temporary if the body's defensive mechanisms are effective. A local infection may persist and spread by extension to become an acute, subacute, or chronic clinical infection or disease state. A local infection may also become systemic when the microorganisms gain access to the lymphatic or vascular system. 2. An infectious disease. [EU]

Infiltration: The diffusion or accumulation in a tissue or cells of substances not normal to it or in amounts of the normal. Also, the material so accumulated. [EU]

Inflammation: A pathological process characterized by injury or destruction of tissues caused by a variety of cytologic and chemical reactions. It is usually manifested by typical signs of pain, heat, redness, swelling, and loss of function. [NIH]

Infusion: A method of putting fluids, including drugs, into the bloodstream. Also called intravenous infusion. [NIH]

Ingestion: Taking into the body by mouth [NIH]

Inhalation: The drawing of air or other substances into the lungs. [EU]

Inner ear: The labyrinth, comprising the vestibule, cochlea, and semicircular canals. [NIH]

Innervation: 1. The distribution or supply of nerves to a part. 2. The supply of nervous energy or of nerve stimulus sent to a part. [EU]

Inorganic: Pertaining to substances not of organic origin. [EU]

Insomnia: Difficulty in going to sleep or getting enough sleep. [NIH]

Intermittent: Occurring at separated intervals; having periods of cessation of activity. [EU]

Intestinal: Having to do with the intestines. [NIH]

Intestine: A long, tube-shaped organ in the abdomen that completes the process of digestion. There is both a large intestine and a small intestine. Also called the bowel. [NIH]

Intoxication: Poisoning, the state of being poisoned. [EU]

Intracellular: Inside a cell. [NIH]

Intracranial Hypertension: Increased pressure within the cranial vault. This may result from several conditions, including hydrocephalus; brain edema; intracranial masses; severe systemic hypertension; pseudotumor cerebri; and other disorders. [NIH]

Intravenous: IV. Into a vein. [NIH]

Intrinsic: Situated entirely within or pertaining exclusively to a part. [EU]

Iodipamide: A water-soluble radiographic contrast media for cholecystography and intravenous cholangiography. [NIH]

Ionizing: Radiation comprising charged particles, e. g. electrons, protons, alpha-particles, etc., having sufficient kinetic energy to produce ionization by collision. [NIH]

Ions: An atom or group of atoms that have a positive or negative electric charge due to a gain (negative charge) or loss (positive charge) of one or more electrons. Atoms with a positive charge are known as cations; those with a negative charge are anions. [NIH]

Isopropyl: A gene mutation inducer. [NIH]

Kb: A measure of the length of DNA fragments, 1 Kb = 1000 base pairs. The largest DNA fragments are up to 50 kilobases long. [NIH]

Keratitis: Inflammation of the cornea. [NIH]

Ketamine: A cyclohexanone derivative used for induction of anesthesia. Its mechanism of action is not well understood, but ketamine can block NMDA receptors (receptors, N-Methyl-D-Aspartate) and may interact with sigma receptors. [NIH]

Kinetics: The study of rate dynamics in chemical or physical systems. [NIH]

Labyrinth: The internal ear; the essential part of the organ of hearing. It consists of an osseous and a membranous portion. [NIH]

Labyrinthine: A vestibular nystagmus resulting from stimulation, injury, or disease of the labyrinth. [NIH]

Laceration: 1. The act of tearing. 2. A torn, ragged, mangled wound. [EU]

Large Intestine: The part of the intestine that goes from the cecum to the rectum. The large intestine absorbs water from stool and changes it from a liquid to a solid form. The large intestine is 5 feet long and includes the appendix, cecum, colon, and rectum. Also called colon. [NIH]

Latency: The period of apparent inactivity between the time when a stimulus is presented and the moment a response occurs. [NIH]

Latent: Phoria which occurs at one distance or another and which usually has no troublesome effect. [NIH]

Latent period: A seemingly inactive period, as that between exposure of tissue to an injurious agent and the manifestation of response, or that between the instant of stimulation and the beginning of response. [EU]

Lesion: An area of abnormal tissue change. [NIH]

Levo: It is an experimental treatment for heroin addiction that was developed by German scientists around 1948 as an analgesic. Like methadone, it binds with opioid receptors, but it is longer acting. [NIH]

Levorphanol: A narcotic analgesic that may be habit-forming. It is nearly as effective orally as by injection. [NIH]

Lidocaine: A local anesthetic and cardiac depressant used as an antiarrhythmia agent. Its actions are more intense and its effects more prolonged than those of procaine but its duration of action is shorter than that of bupivacaine or prilocaine. [NIH]

Ligands: A RNA simulation method developed by the MIT. [NIH]

Lipid: Fat. [NIH]

Liver: A large, glandular organ located in the upper abdomen. The liver cleanses the blood and aids in digestion by secreting bile. [NIH]

Liver Mitochondria: Yellow discoloration of the liver due to fatty degeneration of liver parenchymal cells; the cause may be chemical poisoning. [NIH]

Loa: A genus of parasitic nematodes found throughout the rain-forest areas of the Sudan and the basin of the Congo. L. loa inhabits the subcutaneous tissues, which it traverses freely. [NIH]

Localization: The process of determining or marking the location or site of a lesion or disease. May also refer to the process of keeping a lesion or disease in a specific location or site. [NIH]

Localized: Cancer which has not metastasized yet. [NIH]

Locomotion: Movement or the ability to move from one place or another. It can refer to humans, vertebrate or invertebrate animals, and microorganisms. [NIH]

Long-Term Care: Care over an extended period, usually for a chronic condition or disability, requiring periodic, intermittent, or continuous care. [NIH]

Loratadine: A second-generation histamine H1 receptor antagonist used in the treatment of allergic rhinitis and urticaria. Unlike most classical antihistamines it lacks central nervous system depressing effects such as drowsiness. [NIH]

Lorazepam: An anti-anxiety agent with few side effects. It also has hypnotic, anticonvulsant, and considerable sedative properties and has been proposed as a preanesthetic agent. [NIH]

Lubricants: Oily or slippery substances. [NIH]

Lumbar: Pertaining to the loins, the part of the back between the thorax and the pelvis. [EU]

Lymph: The almost colorless fluid that travels through the lymphatic system and carries cells that help fight infection and disease. [NIH]

Lymph node: A rounded mass of lymphatic tissue that is surrounded by a capsule of connective tissue. Also known as a lymph gland. Lymph nodes are spread out along lymphatic vessels and contain many lymphocytes, which filter the lymphatic fluid (lymph). [NIH]

Lymphatic: The tissues and organs, including the bone marrow, spleen, thymus, and lymph nodes, that produce and store cells that fight infection and disease. [NIH]

Malignant: Cancerous; a growth with a tendency to invade and destroy nearby tissue and spread to other parts of the body. [NIH]

Manic: Affected with mania. [EU]

Manic-depressive psychosis: One of a group of psychotic reactions, fundamentally marked by severe mood swings and a tendency to remission and recurrence. [NIH]

Meclizine: A histamine H1 antagonist used in the treatment of motion sickness, vertigo, and nausea during pregnancy and radiation sickness. [NIH]

Mediate: Indirect; accomplished by the aid of an intervening medium. [EU]

Medicament: A medicinal substance or agent. [EU]

MEDLINE: An online database of MEDLARS, the computerized bibliographic Medical Literature Analysis and Retrieval System of the National Library of Medicine. [NIH]

Medullary: Pertaining to the marrow or to any medulla; resembling marrow. [EU]

Mefenamic Acid: A non-steroidal anti-inflammatory agent with analgesic, anti-inflammatory, and antipyretic properties. It is an inhibitor of cyclooxygenase. [NIH]

Meglumine: 1-Deoxy-1-(methylamino)-D-glucitol. A derivative of sorbitol in which the hydroxyl group in position 1 is replaced by a methylamino group. Often used in conjunction with iodinated organic compounds as contrast medium. [NIH]

Membrane: A very thin layer of tissue that covers a surface. [NIH]

Memory: Complex mental function having four distinct phases: (1) memorizing or learning, (2) retention, (3) recall, and (4) recognition. Clinically, it is usually subdivided into immediate, recent, and remote memory. [NIH]

Meninges: The three membranes that cover and protect the brain and spinal cord. [NIH]

Mental: Pertaining to the mind; psychic. 2. (L. mentum chin) pertaining to the chin. [EU]

Mental Disorders: Psychiatric illness or diseases manifested by breakdowns in the adaptational process expressed primarily as abnormalities of thought, feeling, and behavior producing either distress or impairment of function. [NIH]

Meta-Analysis: A quantitative method of combining the results of independent studies (usually drawn from the published literature) and synthesizing summaries and conclusions which may be used to evaluate therapeutic effectiveness, plan new studies, etc., with application chiefly in the areas of research and medicine. [NIH]

Metabolite: Any substance produced by metabolism or by a metabolic process. [EU]

Methanol: A colorless, flammable liquid used in the manufacture of formaldehyde and acetic acid, in chemical synthesis, antifreeze, and as a solvent. Ingestion of methanol is toxic and may cause blindness. [NIH]

Methapyrilene: Histamine H1 antagonist with sedative action used as a hypnotic and in allergies. [NIH]

Methotrexate: An antineoplastic antimetabolite with immunosuppressant properties. It is an inhibitor of dihydrofolate reductase and prevents the formation of tetrahydrofolate, necessary for synthesis of thymidylate, an essential component of DNA. [NIH]

Methylene Blue: A compound consisting of dark green crystals or crystalline powder, having a bronze-like luster. Solutions in water or alcohol have a deep blue color. Methylene blue is used as a bacteriologic stain and as an indicator. It inhibits Guanylate cyclase, and has been used to treat cyanide poisoning and to lower levels of methemoglobin. [NIH]

Methylphenidate: A central nervous system stimulant used most commonly in the treatment of attention-deficit disorders in children and for narcolepsy. Its mechanisms appear to be similar to those of dextroamphetamine. [NIH]

Methylprednisolone: (6 alpha,11 beta)-11,17,21-Trihydroxy-6-methylpregna-1,4-diene-3,2-dione. A prednisolone derivative which has pharmacological actions similar to prednisolone. [NIH]

Metoclopramide: A dopamine D2 antagonist that is used as an antiemetic. [NIH]

Metoprolol: Adrenergic beta-1-blocking agent with no stimulatory action. It is less bound to plasma albumin than alprenolol and may be useful in angina pectoris, hypertension, or cardiac arrhythmias. [NIH]

Microbe: An organism which cannot be observed with the naked eye; e. g. unicellular animals, lower algae, lower fungi, bacteria. [NIH]

Milligram: A measure of weight. A milligram is approximately 450,000-times smaller than a pound and 28,000-times smaller than an ounce. [NIH]

Modulator: A specific inductor that brings out characteristics peculiar to a definite region. [EU]

Molecular: Of, pertaining to, or composed of molecules : a very small mass of matter. [EU]

Molecular Structure: The location of the atoms, groups or ions relative to one another in a molecule, as well as the number, type and location of covalent bonds. [NIH]

Molecule: A chemical made up of two or more atoms. The atoms in a molecule can be the same (an oxygen molecule has two oxygen atoms) or different (a water molecule has two hydrogen atoms and one oxygen atom). Biological molecules, such as proteins and DNA, can be made up of many thousands of atoms. [NIH]

Morphine: The principal alkaloid in opium and the prototype opiate analgesic and narcotic. Morphine has widespread effects in the central nervous system and on smooth muscle. [NIH]

Motion Sickness: Sickness caused by motion, as sea sickness, train sickness, car sickness, and air sickness. [NIH]

Motor Activity: The physical activity of an organism as a behavioral phenomenon. [NIH]

Mucins: A secretion containing mucopolysaccharides and protein that is the chief constituent of mucus. [NIH]

Mucociliary: Pertaining to or affecting the mucus membrane and hairs (including eyelashes, nose hair, .): mucociliary clearing: the clearance of mucus by ciliary movement (particularly in the respiratory system). [EU]

Mucocutaneous: Pertaining to or affecting the mucous membrane and the skin. [EU]

Mucosa: A mucous membrane, or tunica mucosa. [EU]

Mucositis: A complication of some cancer therapies in which the lining of the digestive system becomes inflamed. Often seen as sores in the mouth. [NIH]

Mucus: The viscous secretion of mucous membranes. It contains mucin, white blood cells, water, inorganic salts, and exfoliated cells. [NIH]

Muscarinic Agonists: Drugs that bind to and activate muscarinic cholinergic receptors (receptors, muscarinic). Muscarinic agonists are most commonly used when it is desirable to increase smooth muscle tone, especially in the GI tract, urinary bladder and the eye. They may also be used to reduce heart rate. [NIH]

Muscle Relaxation: That phase of a muscle twitch during which a muscle returns to a resting position. [NIH]

Mydriatic: 1. Dilating the pupil. 2. Any drug that dilates the pupil. [EU]

Naproxen: An anti-inflammatory agent with analgesic and antipyretic properties. Both the acid and its sodium salt are used in the treatment of rheumatoid arthritis and other rheumatic or musculoskeletal disorders, dysmenorrhea, and acute gout. [NIH]

Narcolepsy: A condition of unknown cause characterized by a periodic uncontrollable tendency to fall asleep. [NIH]

Narcosis: A general and nonspecific reversible depression of neuronal excitability, produced by a number of physical and chemical aspects, usually resulting in stupor. [NIH]

Narcotic: 1. Pertaining to or producing narcosis. 2. An agent that produces insensibility or stupor, applied especially to the opioids, i.e. to any natural or synthetic drug that has morphine-like actions. [EU]

Nausea: An unpleasant sensation in the stomach usually accompanied by the urge to vomit. Common causes are early pregnancy, sea and motion sickness, emotional stress, intense pain, food poisoning, and various enteroviruses. [NIH]

NCI: National Cancer Institute. NCI, part of the National Institutes of Health of the United States Department of Health and Human Services, is the federal government's principal agency for cancer research. NCI conducts, coordinates, and funds cancer research, training, health information dissemination, and other programs with respect to the cause, diagnosis, prevention, and treatment of cancer. Access the NCI Web site at http://cancer.gov. [NIH]

Necrosis: A pathological process caused by the progressive degradative action of enzymes that is generally associated with severe cellular trauma. It is characterized by mitochondrial swelling, nuclear flocculation, uncontrolled cell lysis, and ultimately cell death. [NIH]

Neoplasms: New abnormal growth of tissue. Malignant neoplasms show a greater degree of anaplasia and have the properties of invasion and metastasis, compared to benign neoplasms. [NIH]

Nerve Endings: Specialized terminations of peripheral neurons. Nerve endings include neuroeffector junction(s) by which neurons activate target organs and sensory receptors which transduce information from the various sensory modalities and send it centrally in the nervous system. Presynaptic nerve endings are presynaptic terminals. [NIH]

Nervous System: The entire nerve apparatus composed of the brain, spinal cord, nerves and ganglia. [NIH]

Nervousness: Excessive excitability and irritability, with mental and physical unrest. [EU]

Neurodegenerative Diseases: Hereditary and sporadic conditions which are characterized by progressive nervous system dysfunction. These disorders are often associated with atrophy of the affected central or peripheral nervous system structures. [NIH]

Neuroeffector Junction: The synapse between a neuron (presynaptic) and an effector cell other than another neuron (postsynaptic). Neuroeffector junctions include synapses onto muscles and onto secretory cells. [NIH]

Neuroleptic: A term coined to refer to the effects on cognition and behaviour of antipsychotic drugs, which produce a state of apathy, lack of initiative, and limited range of emotion and in psychotic patients cause a reduction in confusion and agitation and normalization of psychomotor activity. [EU]

Neurologic: Having to do with nerves or the nervous system. [NIH]

Neurology: A medical specialty concerned with the study of the structures, functions, and diseases of the nervous system. [NIH]

Neuromuscular: Pertaining to muscles and nerves. [EU]

Neuromuscular Junction: The synapse between a neuron and a muscle. [NIH]

Neuronal: Pertaining to a neuron or neurons (= conducting cells of the nervous system). [EU]

Neurons: The basic cellular units of nervous tissue. Each neuron consists of a body, an axon, and dendrites. Their purpose is to receive, conduct, and transmit impulses in the nervous system. [NIH]

Neurotoxic: Poisonous or destructive to nerve tissue. [EU]

Neurotoxicity: The tendency of some treatments to cause damage to the nervous system. [NIH]

Neurotransmitter: Any of a group of substances that are released on excitation from the axon terminal of a presynaptic neuron of the central or peripheral nervous system and travel across the synaptic cleft to either excite or inhibit the target cell. Among the many substances that have the properties of a neurotransmitter are acetylcholine, norepinephrine, epinephrine, dopamine, glycine, y-aminobutyrate, glutamic acid, substance P, enkephalins, endorphins, and serotonin. [EU]

Nitrogen: An element with the atomic symbol N, atomic number 7, and atomic weight 14. Nitrogen exists as a diatomic gas and makes up about 78% of the earth's atmosphere by volume. It is a constituent of proteins and nucleic acids and found in all living cells. [NIH]

Nizatidine: A histamine H2 receptor antagonist with low toxicity that inhibits gastric acid secretion. The drug is used for the treatment of duodenal ulcers. [NIH]

Norepinephrine: Precursor of epinephrine that is secreted by the adrenal medulla and is a widespread central and autonomic neurotransmitter. Norepinephrine is the principal transmitter of most postganglionic sympathetic fibers and of the diffuse projection system in the brain arising from the locus ceruleus. It is also found in plants and is used pharmacologically as a sympathomimetic. [NIH]

Nucleic acid: Either of two types of macromolecule (DNA or RNA) formed by polymerization of nucleotides. Nucleic acids are found in all living cells and contain the information (genetic code) for the transfer of genetic information from one generation to the next. [NIH]

Nystagmus: An involuntary, rapid, rhythmic movement of the eyeball, which may be horizontal, vertical, rotatory, or mixed, i.e., of two varieties. [EU]

Ocular: 1. Of, pertaining to, or affecting the eye. 2. Eyepiece. [EU]

Ofloxacin: An orally administered broad-spectrum quinolone antibacterial drug active against most gram-negative and gram-positive bacteria. [NIH]

Ointments: Semisolid preparations used topically for protective emollient effects or as a vehicle for local administration of medications. Ointment bases are various mixtures of fats, waxes, animal and plant oils and solid and liquid hydrocarbons. [NIH]

Ondansetron: A competitive serotonin type 3 receptor antagonist. It is effective in the treatment of nausea and vomiting caused by cytotoxic chemotherapy drugs, including cisplatin, and it has reported anxiolytic and neuroleptic properties. [NIH]

Opiate: A remedy containing or derived from opium; also any drug that induces sleep. [EU]

Opium: The air-dried exudate from the unripe seed capsule of the opium poppy, Papaver somniferum, or its variant, P. album. It contains a number of alkaloids, but only a few - morphine, codeine, and papaverine - have clinical significance. Opium has been used as an analgesic, antitussive, antidiarrheal, and antispasmodic. [NIH]

Optic Nerve: The 2nd cranial nerve. The optic nerve conveys visual information from the retina to the brain. The nerve carries the axons of the retinal ganglion cells which sort at the optic chiasm and continue via the optic tracts to the brain. The largest projection is to the lateral geniculate nuclei; other important targets include the superior colliculi and the suprachiasmatic nuclei. Though known as the second cranial nerve, it is considered part of the central nervous system. [NIH]

Oral Surgical Procedures: Procedures used to treat disease, injuries, and defects of the oral and maxillofacial region. [NIH]

Osteoarthritis: A progressive, degenerative joint disease, the most common form of arthritis, especially in older persons. The disease is thought to result not from the aging process but from biochemical changes and biomechanical stresses affecting articular cartilage. In the foreign literature it is often called osteoarthrosis deformans. [NIH]

Ototoxic: Having a deleterious effect upon the eighth nerve, or upon the organs of hearing and balance. [EU]

Overdosage: 1. The administration of an excessive dose. 2. The condition resulting from an excessive dose. [EU]

Overdose: An accidental or deliberate dose of a medication or street drug that is in excess of what is normally used. [NIH]

Oxazepam: A benzodiazepine used in the treatment of anxiety, alcohol withdrawal, and insomnia. [NIH]

Palate: The structure that forms the roof of the mouth. It consists of the anterior hard palate and the posterior soft palate. [NIH]

Palliative: 1. Affording relief, but not cure. 2. An alleviating medicine. [EU]

Paranasal Sinuses: Air-filled extensions of the respiratory part of the nasal cavity into the frontal, ethmoid, sphenoid, and maxillary cranial bones. They vary in size and form in different individuals and are lined by the ciliated mucous membranes of the nasal cavity. [NIH]

Parkinsonism: A group of neurological disorders characterized by hypokinesia, tremor, and muscular rigidity. [EU]

Paroxysmal: Recurring in paroxysms (= spasms or seizures). [EU]

Partial remission: The shrinking, but not complete disappearance, of a tumor in response to therapy. Also called partial response. [NIH]

Patch: A piece of material used to cover or protect a wound, an injured part, etc.: a patch over the eye. [NIH]

Pathologic: 1. Indicative of or caused by a morbid condition. 2. Pertaining to pathology (= branch of medicine that treats the essential nature of the disease, especially the structural and functional changes in tissues and organs of the body caused by the disease). [EU]

Patient Compliance: Voluntary cooperation of the patient in following a prescribed regimen. [NIH]

Pemphigus: Group of chronic blistering diseases characterized histologically by acantholysis and blister formation within the epidermis. [NIH]

Penicillin: An antibiotic drug used to treat infection. [NIH]

Pepsin: An enzyme made in the stomach that breaks down proteins. [NIH]

Pepsin A: Formed from pig pepsinogen by cleavage of one peptide bond. The enzyme is a single polypeptide chain and is inhibited by methyl 2-diaazoacetamidohexanoate. It cleaves peptides preferentially at the carbonyl linkages of phenylalanine or leucine and acts as the principal digestive enzyme of gastric juice. [NIH]

Peptic: Pertaining to pepsin or to digestion; related to the action of gastric juices. [EU]

Peptide: Any compound consisting of two or more amino acids, the building blocks of proteins. Peptides are combined to make proteins. [NIH]

Perennial: Lasting through the year of for several years. [EU]

Perinatal: Pertaining to or occurring in the period shortly before and after birth; variously defined as beginning with completion of the twentieth to twenty-eighth week of gestation and ending 7 to 28 days after birth. [EU]

Periodontal disease: Disease involving the supporting structures of the teeth (as the gums and periodontal membranes). [NIH]

Periodontal disease: Disease involving the supporting structures of the teeth (as the gums and periodontal membranes). [NIH]

Peripheral Nervous System: The nervous system outside of the brain and spinal cord. The peripheral nervous system has autonomic and somatic divisions. The autonomic nervous system includes the enteric, parasympathetic, and sympathetic subdivisions. The somatic nervous system includes the cranial and spinal nerves and their ganglia and the peripheral sensory receptors. [NIH]

Peritoneum: Endothelial lining of the abdominal cavity, the parietal peritoneum covering the inside of the abdominal wall and the visceral peritoneum covering the bowel, the mesentery, and certain of the organs. The portion that covers the bowel becomes the serosal layer of the bowel wall. [NIH]

Peritonitis: Inflammation of the peritoneum; a condition marked by exudations in the peritoneum of serum, fibrin, cells, and pus. It is attended by abdominal pain and tenderness, constipation, vomiting, and moderate fever. [EU]

Perphenazine: An antipsychotic phenothiazine derivative with actions and uses similar to those of chlorpromazine. [NIH]

Perspiration: Sweating; the functional secretion of sweat. [EU]

Pertussis: An acute, highly contagious infection of the respiratory tract, most frequently affecting young children, usually caused by Bordetella pertussis; a similar illness has been associated with infection by B. parapertussis and B. bronchiseptica. It is characterized by a catarrhal stage, beginning after an incubation period of about two weeks, with slight fever, sneezing, running at the nose, and a dry cough. In a week or two the paroxysmal stage begins, with the characteristic paroxysmal cough, consisting of a deep inspiration, followed by a series of quick, short coughs, continuing until the air is expelled from the lungs; the close of the paroxysm is marked by a long-drawn, shrill, whooping inspiration, due to spasmodic closure of the glottis. This stage lasts three to four weeks, after which the convalescent stage begins, in which paroxysms grow less frequent and less violent, and finally cease. Called also whooping cough. [EU]

Pharmaceutical Preparations: Drugs intended for human or veterinary use, presented in their finished dosage form. Included here are materials used in the preparation and/or formulation of the finished dosage form. [NIH]

Pharmaceutical Solutions: Homogeneous liquid preparations that contain one or more chemical substances dissolved, i.e., molecularly dispersed, in a suitable solvent or mixture of mutually miscible solvents. For reasons of their ingredients, method of preparation, or use, they do not fall into another group of products. [NIH]

Pharmacodynamic: Is concerned with the response of living tissues to chemical stimuli, that is, the action of drugs on the living organism in the absence of disease. [NIH]

Pharmacokinetic: The mathematical analysis of the time courses of absorption, distribution, and elimination of drugs. [NIH]

Pharmacologic: Pertaining to pharmacology or to the properties and reactions of drugs. [EU]

Pharynx: The hollow tube about 5 inches long that starts behind the nose and ends at the top of the trachea (windpipe) and esophagus (the tube that goes to the stomach). [NIH]

Phencyclidine: A hallucinogen formerly used as a veterinary anesthetic, and briefly as a general anesthetic for humans. Phencyclidine is similar to ketamine in structure and in many of its effects. Like ketamine, it can produce a dissociative state. It exerts its pharmacological action through inhibition of NMDA receptors (receptors, N-methyl-D-aspartate). As a drug of abuse, it is known as PCP and Angel Dust. [NIH]

Phenytoin: An anticonvulsant that is used in a wide variety of seizures. It is also an anti-arrhythmic and a muscle relaxant. The mechanism of therapeutic action is not clear, although several cellular actions have been described including effects on ion channels, active transport, and general membrane stabilization. The mechanism of its muscle relaxant effect appears to involve a reduction in the sensitivity of muscle spindles to stretch. Phenytoin has been proposed for several other therapeutic uses, but its use has been limited by its many adverse effects and interactions with other drugs. [NIH]

Phlebitis: Inflammation of a vein. [NIH]

Phosphorus: A non-metallic element that is found in the blood, muscles, nevers, bones, and teeth, and is a component of adenosine triphosphate (ATP; the primary energy source for the body's cells.) [NIH]

Photoallergy: Sensitization of the skin to light usually due to the action of certain substances or drugs, may occur shortly after exposure to a substance or after a latent period of from days to months. [NIH]

Photocoagulation: Using a special strong beam of light (laser) to seal off bleeding blood vessels such as in the eye. The laser can also burn away blood vessels that should not have grown in the eye. This is the main treatment for diabetic retinopathy. [NIH]

Photodynamic therapy: Treatment with drugs that become active when exposed to light. These drugs kill cancer cells. [NIH]

Physiologic: Having to do with the functions of the body. When used in the phrase "physiologic age," it refers to an age assigned by general health, as opposed to calendar age. [NIH]

Physostigmine: A cholinesterase inhibitor that is rapidly absorbed through membranes. It can be applied topically to the conjunctiva. It also can cross the blood-brain barrier and is used when central nervous system effects are desired, as in the treatment of severe anticholinergic toxicity. [NIH]

Pilot study: The initial study examining a new method or treatment. [NIH]

Piroxicam: 4-Hydroxy-2-methyl-N-2-pyridyl-2H-1,2-benzothiazine-3-carboxamide 1,1-dioxide. A non-steroidal anti-inflammatory agent that is well established in the treatment of rheumatoid arthritis and osteoarthritis. Its usefulness has also been demonstrated in the treatment of musculoskeletal disorders, dysmenorrhea, and postoperative pain. Its long half-life enables it to be administered once daily. The drug has also been shown to be effective if administered rectally. Gastrointestinal complaints are the most frequently reported side effects. [NIH]

Plants: Multicellular, eukaryotic life forms of the kingdom Plantae. They are characterized by a mainly photosynthetic mode of nutrition; essentially unlimited growth at localized regions of cell divisions (meristems); cellulose within cells providing rigidity; the absence of organs of locomotion; absense of nervous and sensory systems; and an alteration of haploid and diploid generations. [NIH]

Plasma: The clear, yellowish, fluid part of the blood that carries the blood cells. The proteins that form blood clots are in plasma. [NIH]

Plasma protein: One of the hundreds of different proteins present in blood plasma, including carrier proteins (such albumin, transferrin, and haptoglobin), fibrinogen and other coagulation factors, complement components, immunoglobulins, enzyme inhibitors, precursors of substances such as angiotension and bradykinin, and many other types of proteins. [EU]

Platelet Transfusion: The transfer of blood platelets from a donor to a recipient or reinfusion to the donor. [NIH]

Pneumonia: Inflammation of the lungs. [NIH]

Poisoning: A condition or physical state produced by the ingestion, injection or inhalation of, or exposure to a deleterious agent. [NIH]

Pollen: The male fertilizing element of flowering plants analogous to sperm in animals. It is released from the anthers as yellow dust, to be carried by insect or other vectors, including wind, to the ovary (stigma) of other flowers to produce the embryo enclosed by the seed. The pollens of many plants are allergenic. [NIH]

Polypeptide: A peptide which on hydrolysis yields more than two amino acids; called tripeptides, tetrapeptides, etc. according to the number of amino acids contained. [EU]

Posterior: Situated in back of, or in the back part of, or affecting the back or dorsal surface of the body. In lower animals, it refers to the caudal end of the body. [EU]

Postoperative: After surgery. [NIH]

Potassium: An element that is in the alkali group of metals. It has an atomic symbol K, atomic number 19, and atomic weight 39.10. It is the chief cation in the intracellular fluid of muscle and other cells. Potassium ion is a strong electrolyte and it plays a significant role in the regulation of fluid volume and maintenance of the water-electrolyte balance. [NIH]

Potentiating: A degree of synergism which causes the exposure of the organism to a harmful substance to worsen a disease already contracted. [NIH]

Practice Guidelines: Directions or principles presenting current or future rules of policy for the health care practitioner to assist him in patient care decisions regarding diagnosis, therapy, or related clinical circumstances. The guidelines may be developed by government agencies at any level, institutions, professional societies, governing boards, or by the convening of expert panels. The guidelines form a basis for the evaluation of all aspects of health care and delivery. [NIH]

Precursor: Something that precedes. In biological processes, a substance from which another, usually more active or mature substance is formed. In clinical medicine, a sign or symptom that heralds another. [EU]

Prednisolone: A glucocorticoid with the general properties of the corticosteroids. It is the drug of choice for all conditions in which routine systemic corticosteroid therapy is indicated, except adrenal deficiency states. [NIH]

Prednisone: A synthetic anti-inflammatory glucocorticoid derived from cortisone. It is biologically inert and converted to prednisolone in the liver. [NIH]

Premedication: Preliminary administration of a drug preceding a diagnostic, therapeutic, or surgical procedure. The commonest types of premedication are antibiotics (antibiotic prophylaxis) and anti-anxiety agents. It does not include preanesthetic medication. [NIH]

Presynaptic: Situated proximal to a synapse, or occurring before the synapse is crossed. [EU]

Presynaptic Terminals: The distal terminations of axons which are specialized for the release of neurotransmitters. Also included are varicosities along the course of axons which have similar specializations and also release transmitters. Presynaptic terminals in both the central and peripheral nervous systems are included. [NIH]

Procaine: A local anesthetic of the ester type that has a slow onset and a short duration of action. It is mainly used for infiltration anesthesia, peripheral nerve block, and spinal block. (From Martindale, The Extra Pharmacopoeia, 30th ed, p1016). [NIH]

Procyclidine: A muscarinic antagonist that crosses the blood-brain barrier and is used in the treatment of drug-induced extrapyramidal disorders and in parkinsonism. [NIH]

Progenitalis: A group of acute infections causes by herpes simplex virus type 1 or type 2, characterized by the development of one or more small fluid-filled vesicles with a raised erythematous base on the skin or mucous membrane, and occurring as a primary infection or recurring because of reactivation of a latent infection. Type 1 infections usually involve nongenital regions of the body, whereas in type 2 infections the lesions are primarily seen on the genital and surrounding areas. Precipitating factors include fever, exposure to cold temperature or to ultraviolet rays, sunburn, cutaneous or mucosal abrasions, emotional stress, and nerve injury. [EU]

Progressive: Advancing; going forward; going from bad to worse; increasing in scope or severity. [EU]

Promethazine: A phenothiazine derivative with histamine H1-blocking, antimuscarinic, and sedative properties. It is used as an antiallergic, in pruritus, for motion sickness and sedation, and also in animals. [NIH]

Prone: Having the front portion of the body downwards. [NIH]

Propolis: Resinous substance obtained from beehives; contains many different substances which may have antimicrobial or antimycotic activity topically; its extracts are called propolis resin or balsam. Synonyms: bee bread; hive dross; bee glue. [NIH]

Propoxyphene: A narcotic analgesic structurally related to methadone. Only the dextro-isomer has an analgesic effect; the levo-isomer appears to exert an antitussive effect. [NIH]

Propylene Glycol: A clear, colorless, viscous organic solvent and diluent used in pharmaceutical preparations. [NIH]

Protective Agents: Synthetic or natural substances which are given to prevent a disease or disorder or are used in the process of treating a disease or injury due to a poisonous agent. [NIH]

Protein S: The vitamin K-dependent cofactor of activated protein C. Together with protein C, it inhibits the action of factors VIIIa and Va. A deficiency in protein S can lead to recurrent venous and arterial thrombosis. [NIH]

Proteins: Polymers of amino acids linked by peptide bonds. The specific sequence of amino acids determines the shape and function of the protein. [NIH]

Protons: Stable elementary particles having the smallest known positive charge, found in the nuclei of all elements. The proton mass is less than that of a neutron. A proton is the nucleus of the light hydrogen atom, i.e., the hydrogen ion. [NIH]

Proximal: Nearest; closer to any point of reference; opposed to distal. [EU]

Proxy: A person authorized to decide or act for another person, for example, a person having durable power of attorney. [NIH]

Pruritus: An intense itching sensation that produces the urge to rub or scratch the skin to obtain relief. [NIH]

Psychiatric: Pertaining to or within the purview of psychiatry. [EU]

Psychiatry: The medical science that deals with the origin, diagnosis, prevention, and treatment of mental disorders. [NIH]

Psychic: Pertaining to the psyche or to the mind; mental. [EU]

Psychoactive: Those drugs which alter sensation, mood, consciousness or other psychological or behavioral functions. [NIH]

Psychomotor Performance: The coordination of a sensory or ideational (cognitive) process and a motor activity. [NIH]

Psychophysiology: The study of the physiological basis of human and animal behavior. [NIH]

Psychosis: A mental disorder characterized by gross impairment in reality testing as evidenced by delusions, hallucinations, markedly incoherent speech, or disorganized and agitated behaviour without apparent awareness on the part of the patient of the incomprehensibility of his behaviour; the term is also used in a more general sense to refer to mental disorders in which mental functioning is sufficiently impaired as to interfere grossly with the patient's capacity to meet the ordinary demands of life. Historically, the term has been applied to many conditions, e.g. manic-depressive psychosis, that were first described in psychotic patients, although many patients with the disorder are not judged psychotic. [EU]

Public Policy: A course or method of action selected, usually by a government, from among alternatives to guide and determine present and future decisions. [NIH]

Publishing: "The business or profession of the commercial production and issuance of literature" (Webster's 3d). It includes the publisher, publication processes, editing and editors. Production may be by conventional printing methods or by electronic publishing. [NIH]

Pulmonary: Relating to the lungs. [NIH]

Pulmonary Edema: An accumulation of an excessive amount of watery fluid in the lungs, may be caused by acute exposure to dangerous concentrations of irritant gasses. [NIH]

Purpura: Purplish or brownish red discoloration, easily visible through the epidermis, caused by hemorrhage into the tissues. [NIH]

Pyrilamine: A histamine H1 antagonist. It has mild hypnotic properties and some local anesthetic action and is used for allergies (including skin eruptions) both parenterally and locally. It is a common ingredient of cold remedies. [NIH]

Quaternary: 1. Fourth in order. 2. Containing four elements or groups. [EU]

Radiation: Emission or propagation of electromagnetic energy (waves/rays), or the waves/rays themselves; a stream of electromagnetic particles (electrons, neutrons, protons, alpha particles) or a mixture of these. The most common source is the sun. [NIH]

Radiation therapy: The use of high-energy radiation from x-rays, gamma rays, neutrons, and other sources to kill cancer cells and shrink tumors. Radiation may come from a machine outside the body (external-beam radiation therapy), or it may come from radioactive material placed in the body in the area near cancer cells (internal radiation therapy, implant radiation, or brachytherapy). Systemic radiation therapy uses a radioactive substance, such as a radiolabeled monoclonal antibody, that circulates throughout the body. Also called radiotherapy. [NIH]

Radioactive: Giving off radiation. [NIH]

Radiography: Examination of any part of the body for diagnostic purposes by means of roentgen rays, recording the image on a sensitized surface (such as photographic film). [NIH]

Radioimmunotherapy: Radiotherapy where cytotoxic radionuclides are linked to antibodies in order to deliver toxins directly to tumor targets. Therapy with targeted radiation rather than antibody-targeted toxins (immunotoxins) has the advantage that adjacent tumor cells, which lack the appropriate antigenic determinants, can be destroyed by radiation cross-fire. Radioimmunotherapy is sometimes called targeted radiotherapy, but this latter term can also refer to radionuclides linked to non-immune molecules (radiotherapy). [NIH]

Radiotherapy: The use of ionizing radiation to treat malignant neoplasms and other benign conditions. The most common forms of ionizing radiation used as therapy are x-rays, gamma rays, and electrons. A special form of radiotherapy, targeted radiotherapy, links a cytotoxic radionuclide to a molecule that targets the tumor. When this molecule is an antibody or other immunologic molecule, the technique is called radioimmunotherapy. [NIH]

Randomized: Describes an experiment or clinical trial in which animal or human subjects are assigned by chance to separate groups that compare different treatments. [NIH]

Ranitidine: A non-imidazole blocker of those histamine receptors that mediate gastric secretion (H2 receptors). It is used to treat gastrointestinal ulcers. [NIH]

Ranitidine Hydrochloride: Drug used to eradicate Helicobacter pylori. [NIH]

Reactivation: The restoration of activity to something that has been inactivated. [EU]

Reagent: A substance employed to produce a chemical reaction so as to detect, measure, produce, etc., other substances. [EU]

Reality Testing: The individual's objective evaluation of the external world and the ability to differentiate adequately between it and the internal world; considered to be a primary ego function. [NIH]

Receptor: A molecule inside or on the surface of a cell that binds to a specific substance and causes a specific physiologic effect in the cell. [NIH]

Rectal: By or having to do with the rectum. The rectum is the last 8 to 10 inches of the large intestine and ends at the anus. [NIH]

Rectum: The last 8 to 10 inches of the large intestine. [NIH]

Red Nucleus: A pinkish-yellow portion of the midbrain situated in the rostral mesencephalic tegmentum. It receives a large projection from the contralateral half of the cerebellum via the superior cerebellar peduncle and a projection from the ipsilateral motor cortex. [NIH]

Reductase: Enzyme converting testosterone to dihydrotestosterone. [NIH]

Refer: To send or direct for treatment, aid, information, de decision. [NIH]

Reflex: An involuntary movement or exercise of function in a part, excited in response to a stimulus applied to the periphery and transmitted to the brain or spinal cord. [NIH]

Reflux: The term used when liquid backs up into the esophagus from the stomach. [NIH]

Refractory: Not readily yielding to treatment. [EU]

Refractory cancer: Cancer that has not responded to treatment. [NIH]

Regimen: A treatment plan that specifies the dosage, the schedule, and the duration of treatment. [NIH]

Regurgitation: A backward flowing, as the casting up of undigested food, or the backward flowing of blood into the heart, or between the chambers of the heart when a valve is incompetent. [EU]

Remission: A decrease in or disappearance of signs and symptoms of cancer. In partial remission, some, but not all, signs and symptoms of cancer have disappeared. In complete remission, all signs and symptoms of cancer have disappeared, although there still may be cancer in the body. [NIH]

Renal failure: Progressive renal insufficiency and uremia, due to irreversible and progressive renal glomerular tubular or interstitial disease. [NIH]

Research Design: A plan for collecting and utilizing data so that desired information can be obtained with sufficient precision or so that an hypothesis can be tested properly. [NIH]

Reserpine: An alkaloid found in the roots of Rauwolfia serpentina and R. vomitoria. Reserpine inhibits the uptake of norepinephrine into storage vesicles resulting in depletion of catecholamines and serotonin from central and peripheral axon terminals. It has been used as an antihypertensive and an antipsychotic as well as a research tool, but its adverse effects limit its clinical use. [NIH]

Resorption: The loss of substance through physiologic or pathologic means, such as loss of dentin and cementum of a tooth, or of the alveolar process of the mandible or maxilla. [EU]

Respiratory distress syndrome: A lung disease that occurs primarily in premature infants; the newborn must struggle for each breath and blueing of its skin reflects the baby's inability to get enough oxygen. [NIH]

Respiratory Physiology: Functions and activities of the respiratory tract as a whole or of any of its parts. [NIH]

Retina: The ten-layered nervous tissue membrane of the eye. It is continuous with the optic nerve and receives images of external objects and transmits visual impulses to the brain. Its outer surface is in contact with the choroid and the inner surface with the vitreous body. The outer-most layer is pigmented, whereas the inner nine layers are transparent. [NIH]

Rheumatoid: Resembling rheumatism. [EU]

Rheumatoid arthritis: A form of arthritis, the cause of which is unknown, although infection, hypersensitivity, hormone imbalance and psychologic stress have been suggested as possible causes. [NIH]

Rhinitis: Inflammation of the mucous membrane of the nose. [NIH]

Rigidity: Stiffness or inflexibility, chiefly that which is abnormal or morbid; rigor. [EU]

Ristocetin: An antibiotic mixture of two components, A and B, obtained from Nocardia lurida (or the same substance produced by any other means). It is no longer used clinically because of its toxicity. It causes platelet agglutination and blood coagulation and is used to assay those functions in vitro. [NIH]

Rod: A reception for vision, located in the retina. [NIH]

Salicylate: Non-steroidal anti-inflammatory drugs. [NIH]

Saline: A solution of salt and water. [NIH]

Saliva: The clear, viscous fluid secreted by the salivary glands and mucous glands of the mouth. It contains mucins, water, organic salts, and ptylin. [NIH]

Salivary: The duct that convey saliva to the mouth. [NIH]

Salivary glands: Glands in the mouth that produce saliva. [NIH]

Salivation: 1. The secretion of saliva. 2. Ptyalism (= excessive flow of saliva). [EU]

Schizoid: Having qualities resembling those found in greater degree in schizophrenics; a person of schizoid personality. [NIH]

Schizophrenia: A mental disorder characterized by a special type of disintegration of the personality. [NIH]

Schizotypal Personality Disorder: A personality disorder in which there are oddities of thought (magical thinking, paranoid ideation, suspiciousness), perception (illusions, depersonalization), speech (digressive, vague, overelaborate), and behavior (inappropriate affect in social interactions, frequently social isolation) that are not severe enough to characterize schizophrenia. [NIH]

Scopolamine: An alkaloid from Solanaceae, especially Datura metel L. and Scopola carniolica. Scopolamine and its quaternary derivatives act as antimuscarinics like atropine, but may have more central nervous system effects. Among the many uses are as an anesthetic premedication, in urinary incontinence, in motion sickness, as an antispasmodic, and as a mydriatic and cycloplegic. [NIH]

Screening: Checking for disease when there are no symptoms. [NIH]

Sebaceous: Gland that secretes sebum. [NIH]

Secobarbital: A barbiturate that is used as a sedative. Secobarbital is reported to have no anti-anxiety activity. [NIH]

Secretion: 1. The process of elaborating a specific product as a result of the activity of a gland; this activity may range from separating a specific substance of the blood to the elaboration of a new chemical substance. 2. Any substance produced by secretion. [EU]

Sedative: 1. Allaying activity and excitement. 2. An agent that allays excitement. [EU]

Sedatives, Barbiturate: Those derivatives of barbituric or thiobarbituric acid that are used as hypnotics or sedatives. The structural class of all such derivatives, regardless of use, is barbiturates. [NIH]

Sediment: A precipitate, especially one that is formed spontaneously. [EU]

Sedimentation: The act of causing the deposit of sediment, especially by the use of a centrifugal machine. [EU]

Seizures: Clinical or subclinical disturbances of cortical function due to a sudden, abnormal, excessive, and disorganized discharge of brain cells. Clinical manifestations include abnormal motor, sensory and psychic phenomena. Recurrent seizures are usually referred to as epilepsy or "seizure disorder." [NIH]

Self Care: Performance of activities or tasks traditionally performed by professional health care providers. The concept includes care of oneself or one's family and friends. [NIH]

Semicircular canal: Three long canals of the bony labyrinth of the ear, forming loops and opening into the vestibule by five openings. [NIH]

Sensitization: 1. Administration of antigen to induce a primary immune response; priming; immunization. 2. Exposure to allergen that results in the development of hypersensitivity. 3. The coating of erythrocytes with antibody so that they are subject to lysis by complement in the presence of homologous antigen, the first stage of a complement fixation test. [EU]

Serologic: Analysis of a person's serum, especially specific immune or lytic serums. [NIH]

Serotonin: A biochemical messenger and regulator, synthesized from the essential amino acid L-tryptophan. In humans it is found primarily in the central nervous system, gastrointestinal tract, and blood platelets. Serotonin mediates several important physiological functions including neurotransmission, gastrointestinal motility, hemostasis, and cardiovascular integrity. Multiple receptor families (receptors, serotonin) explain the broad physiological actions and distribution of this biochemical mediator. [NIH]

Serum: The clear liquid part of the blood that remains after blood cells and clotting proteins have been removed. [NIH]

Shock: The general bodily disturbance following a severe injury; an emotional or moral upset occasioned by some disturbing or unexpected experience; disruption of the circulation, which can upset all body functions: sometimes referred to as circulatory shock. [NIH]

Side effect: A consequence other than the one(s) for which an agent or measure is used, as the adverse effects produced by a drug, especially on a tissue or organ system other than the one sought to be benefited by its administration. [EU]

Signs and Symptoms: Clinical manifestations that can be either objective when observed by a physician, or subjective when perceived by the patient. [NIH]

Silicon: A trace element that constitutes about 27.6% of the earth's crust in the form of silicon dioxide. It does not occur free in nature. Silicon has the atomic symbol Si, atomic number 14, and atomic weight 28.09. [NIH]

Silicon Dioxide: Silica. Transparent, tasteless crystals found in nature as agate, amethyst, chalcedony, cristobalite, flint, sand, quartz, and tridymite. The compound is insoluble in water or acids except hydrofluoric acid. [NIH]

Sinusitis: An inflammatory process of the mucous membranes of the paranasal sinuses that occurs in three stages: acute, subacute, and chronic. Sinusitis results from any condition causing ostial obstruction or from pathophysiologic changes in the mucociliary transport mechanism. [NIH]

Small intestine: The part of the digestive tract that is located between the stomach and the large intestine. [NIH]

Smooth muscle: Muscle that performs automatic tasks, such as constricting blood vessels. [NIH]

Sneezing: Sudden, forceful, involuntary expulsion of air from the nose and mouth caused by irritation to the mucous membranes of the upper respiratory tract. [NIH]

Sodium: An element that is a member of the alkali group of metals. It has the atomic symbol Na, atomic number 11, and atomic weight 23. With a valence of 1, it has a strong affinity for oxygen and other nonmetallic elements. Sodium provides the chief cation of the extracellular body fluids. Its salts are the most widely used in medicine. (From Dorland, 27th ed) Physiologically the sodium ion plays a major role in blood pressure regulation, maintenance of fluid volume, and electrolyte balance. [NIH]

Sodium Bicarbonate: A white, crystalline powder that is commonly used as a pH buffering agent, an electrolyte replenisher, systemic alkalizer and in topical cleansing solutions. [NIH]

Solvent: 1. Dissolving; effecting a solution. 2. A liquid that dissolves or that is capable of dissolving; the component of a solution that is present in greater amount. [EU]

Soporific: 1. Causing or inducing profound sleep. 2. A drug or other agent which induces sleep. [EU]

Sorbitol: A polyhydric alcohol with about half the sweetness of sucrose. Sorbitol occurs naturally and is also produced synthetically from glucose. It was formerly used as a diuretic and may still be used as a laxative and in irrigating solutions for some surgical procedures. It is also used in many manufacturing processes, as a pharmaceutical aid, and in several research applications. [NIH]

Spasm: An involuntary contraction of a muscle or group of muscles. Spasms may involve skeletal muscle or smooth muscle. [NIH]

Spasmodic: Of the nature of a spasm. [EU]

Specialist: In medicine, one who concentrates on 1 special branch of medical science. [NIH]

Species: A taxonomic category subordinate to a genus (or subgenus) and superior to a subspecies or variety, composed of individuals possessing common characters distinguishing them from other categories of individuals of the same taxonomic level. In taxonomic nomenclature, species are designated by the genus name followed by a Latin or Latinized adjective or noun. [EU]

Specificity: Degree of selectivity shown by an antibody with respect to the number and types of antigens with which the antibody combines, as well as with respect to the rates and the extents of these reactions. [NIH]

Spinal cord: The main trunk or bundle of nerves running down the spine through holes in the spinal bone (the vertebrae) from the brain to the level of the lower back. [NIH]

Spleen: An organ that is part of the lymphatic system. The spleen produces lymphocytes, filters the blood, stores blood cells, and destroys old blood cells. It is located on the left side of the abdomen near the stomach. [NIH]

Sporadic: Neither endemic nor epidemic; occurring occasionally in a random or isolated manner. [EU]

Sterile: Unable to produce children. [NIH]

Sterility: 1. The inability to produce offspring, i.e., the inability to conceive (female s.) or to induce conception (male s.). 2. The state of being aseptic, or free from microorganisms. [EU]

Steroid: A group name for lipids that contain a hydrogenated cyclopentanoperhydrophenanthrene ring system. Some of the substances included in this group are progesterone, adrenocortical hormones, the gonadal hormones, cardiac aglycones, bile acids, sterols (such as cholesterol), toad poisons, saponins, and some of the carcinogenic hydrocarbons. [EU]

Stimulant: 1. Producing stimulation; especially producing stimulation by causing tension on muscle fibre through the nervous tissue. 2. An agent or remedy that produces stimulation. [EU]

Stimulus: That which can elicit or evoke action (response) in a muscle, nerve, gland or other excitable issue, or cause an augmenting action upon any function or metabolic process. [NIH]

Stomach: An organ of digestion situated in the left upper quadrant of the abdomen between the termination of the esophagus and the beginning of the duodenum. [NIH]

Stress: Forcibly exerted influence; pressure. Any condition or situation that causes strain or tension. Stress may be either physical or psychologic, or both. [NIH]

Stroke: Sudden loss of function of part of the brain because of loss of blood flow. Stroke may be caused by a clot (thrombosis) or rupture (hemorrhage) of a blood vessel to the brain. [NIH]

Stupor: Partial or nearly complete unconsciousness, manifested by the subject's responding only to vigorous stimulation. Also, in psychiatry, a disorder marked by reduced responsiveness. [EU]

Subacute: Somewhat acute; between acute and chronic. [EU]

Subarachnoid: Situated or occurring between the arachnoid and the pia mater. [EU]

Subclinical: Without clinical manifestations; said of the early stage(s) of an infection or other disease or abnormality before symptoms and signs become apparent or detectable by clinical examination or laboratory tests, or of a very mild form of an infection or other disease or abnormality. [EU]

Subcutaneous: Beneath the skin. [NIH]

Sublingual: Located beneath the tongue. [EU]

Substance P: An eleven-amino acid neurotransmitter that appears in both the central and peripheral nervous systems. It is involved in transmission of pain, causes rapid contractions of the gastrointestinal smooth muscle, and modulates inflammatory and immune responses. [NIH]

Substrate: A substance upon which an enzyme acts. [EU]

Sucralfate: A basic aluminum complex of sulfated sucrose. It is advocated in the therapy of peptic, duodenal, and prepyloric ulcers, gastritis, reflux esophagitis, and other gastrointestinal irritations. It acts primarily at the ulcer site, where it has cytoprotective, pepsinostatic, antacid, and bile acid-binding properties. The drug is only slightly absorbed by the digestive mucosa, which explains the absence of systemic effects and toxicity. [NIH]

Sulindac: A sulfinylindene derivative whose sulfinyl moiety is converted in vivo to an active anti-inflammatory analgesic that undergoes enterohepatic circulation to maintain constant blood levels without causing gastrointestinal side effects. [NIH]

Surfactant: A fat-containing protein in the respiratory passages which reduces the surface tension of pulmonary fluids and contributes to the elastic properties of pulmonary tissue. [NIH]

Sweat: The fluid excreted by the sweat glands. It consists of water containing sodium chloride, phosphate, urea, ammonia, and other waste products. [NIH]

Sweat Glands: Sweat-producing structures that are embedded in the dermis. Each gland consists of a single tube, a coiled body, and a superficial duct. [NIH]

Sympathomimetic: 1. Mimicking the effects of impulses conveyed by adrenergic postganglionic fibres of the sympathetic nervous system. 2. An agent that produces effects similar to those of impulses conveyed by adrenergic postganglionic fibres of the sympathetic nervous system. Called also adrenergic. [EU]

Symptomatic: Having to do with symptoms, which are signs of a condition or disease. [NIH]

Symptomatic treatment: Therapy that eases symptoms without addressing the cause of disease. [NIH]

Symptomatology: 1. That branch of medicine with treats of symptoms; the systematic discussion of symptoms. 2. The combined symptoms of a disease. [EU]

Synapse: The region where the processes of two neurons come into close contiguity, and the nervous impulse passes from one to the other; the fibers of the two are intermeshed, but, according to the general view, there is no direct contiguity. [NIH]

Systemic: Affecting the entire body. [NIH]

Systemic disease: Disease that affects the whole body. [NIH]

Systolic: Indicating the maximum arterial pressure during contraction of the left ventricle of the heart. [EU]

Tachycardia: Excessive rapidity in the action of the heart, usually with a heart rate above 100 beats per minute. [NIH]

Taste Buds: Small sensory organs which contain gustatory receptor cells, basal cells, and supporting cells. Taste buds in humans are found in the epithelia of the tongue, palate, and pharynx. They are innervated by the chorda tympani nerve (a branch of the facial nerve) and the glossopharyngeal nerve. [NIH]

Temazepam: A benzodiazepinone that acts as a GABA modulator and anti-anxiety agent. [NIH]

Terbutaline: A selective beta-2 adrenergic agonist used as a bronchodilator and tocolytic. [NIH]

Terfenadine: A selective histamine H1-receptor antagonist devoid of central nervous system depressant activity. The drug is used in the treatment of seasonal allergic rhinitis, asthma, allergic conjunctivitis, and chronic idiopathic urticaria. [NIH]

Tetanus: A disease caused by tetanospasmin, a powerful protein toxin produced by Clostridium tetani. Tetanus usually occurs after an acute injury, such as a puncture wound or laceration. Generalized tetanus, the most common form, is characterized by tetanic muscular contractions and hyperreflexia. Localized tetanus presents itself as a mild condition with manifestations restricted to muscles near the wound. It may progress to the generalized form. [NIH]

Thalamic: Cell that reaches the lateral nucleus of amygdala. [NIH]

Thalamic Diseases: Disorders of the centrally located thalamus, which integrates a wide range of cortical and subcortical information. Manifestations include sensory loss, movement disorders; ataxia, pain syndromes, visual disorders, a variety of neuropsychological conditions, and coma. Relatively common etiologies include cerebrovascular disorders; craniocerebral trauma; brain neoplasms; brain hypoxia; intracranial hemorrhages; and infectious processes. [NIH]

Theophylline: Alkaloid obtained from Thea sinensis (tea) and others. It stimulates the heart and central nervous system, dilates bronchi and blood vessels, and causes diuresis. The drug is used mainly in bronchial asthma and for myocardial stimulation. Among its more prominent cellular effects are inhibition of cyclic nucleotide phosphodiesterases and antagonism of adenosine receptors. [NIH]

Therapeutics: The branch of medicine which is concerned with the treatment of diseases, palliative or curative. [NIH]

Thermal: Pertaining to or characterized by heat. [EU]

Thiothixene: A thioxanthine used as an antipsychotic agent. Its effects are similar to the phenothiazine antipsychotics. [NIH]

Thoracic: Having to do with the chest. [NIH]

Threshold: For a specified sensory modality (e. g. light, sound, vibration), the lowest level (absolute threshold) or smallest difference (difference threshold, difference limen) or intensity of the stimulus discernible in prescribed conditions of stimulation. [NIH]

Thrombosis: The formation or presence of a blood clot inside a blood vessel. [NIH]

Thymus: An organ that is part of the lymphatic system, in which T lymphocytes grow and multiply. The thymus is in the chest behind the breastbone. [NIH]

Tinnitus: Sounds that are perceived in the absence of any external noise source which may take the form of buzzing, ringing, clicking, pulsations, and other noises. Objective tinnitus refers to noises generated from within the ear or adjacent structures that can be heard by other individuals. The term subjective tinnitus is used when the sound is audible only to the affected individual. Tinnitus may occur as a manifestation of cochlear diseases; vestibulocochlear nerve diseases; intracranial hypertension; craniocerebral trauma; and other conditions. [NIH]

Tissue: A group or layer of cells that are alike in type and work together to perform a specific function. [NIH]

Tolerance: 1. The ability to endure unusually large doses of a drug or toxin. 2. Acquired drug tolerance; a decreasing response to repeated constant doses of a drug or the need for increasing doses to maintain a constant response. [EU]

Tonic: 1. Producing and restoring the normal tone. 2. Characterized by continuous tension. 3. A term formerly used for a class of medicinal preparations believed to have the power of restoring normal tone to tissue. [EU]

Tonicity: The normal state of muscular tension. [NIH]

Topical: On the surface of the body. [NIH]

Toxic: Having to do with poison or something harmful to the body. Toxic substances usually cause unwanted side effects. [NIH]

Toxicity: The quality of being poisonous, especially the degree of virulence of a toxic microbe or of a poison. [EU]

Toxicology: The science concerned with the detection, chemical composition, and pharmacologic action of toxic substances or poisons and the treatment and prevention of toxic manifestations. [NIH]

Toxin: A poison; frequently used to refer specifically to a protein produced by some higher plants, certain animals, and pathogenic bacteria, which is highly toxic for other living organisms. Such substances are differentiated from the simple chemical poisons and the vegetable alkaloids by their high molecular weight and antigenicity. [EU]

Trace element: Substance or element essential to plant or animal life, but present in extremely small amounts. [NIH]

Transdermal: Entering through the dermis, or skin, as in administration of a drug applied to the skin in ointment or patch form. [EU]

Transfection: The uptake of naked or purified DNA into cells, usually eukaryotic. It is analogous to bacterial transformation. [NIH]

Transmitter: A chemical substance which effects the passage of nerve impulses from one cell to the other at the synapse. [NIH]

Trauma: Any injury, wound, or shock, must frequently physical or structural shock, producing a disturbance. [NIH]

Triazolam: A short-acting benzodiazepine used in the treatment of insomnia. Some countries temporarily withdrew triazolam from the market because of concerns about adverse reactions, mostly psychological, associated with higher dose ranges. Its use at lower doses with appropriate care and labeling has been reaffirmed by the FDA and most other countries. [NIH]

Tricyclic: Containing three fused rings or closed chains in the molecular structure. [EU]

Trihexyphenidyl: A centrally acting muscarinic antagonist used in the treatment of parkinsonism and drug-induced extrapyramidal movement disorders and as an antispasmodic. [NIH]

Tripelennamine: A histamine H1 antagonist with low sedative action but frequent gastrointestinal irritation. It is used to treat asthma, hay fever, urticaria, and rhinitis, and also in veterinary applications. Tripelennamine is administered by various routes, including topically. [NIH]

Trismus: Spasmodic contraction of the masseter muscle resulting in forceful jaw closure. This may be seen with a variety of diseases, including tetanus, as a complication of radiation therapy, trauma, or in association with neoplastic conditions. [NIH]

Ulcer: A localized necrotic lesion of the skin or a mucous surface. [NIH]

Urea: A compound (CO(NH2)2), formed in the liver from ammonia produced by the deamination of amino acids. It is the principal end product of protein catabolism and constitutes about one half of the total urinary solids. [NIH]

Urethra: The tube through which urine leaves the body. It empties urine from the bladder. [NIH]

Uridine Diphosphate: A uracil nucleotide containing a pyrophosphate group esterified to C5 of the sugar moiety. [NIH]

Uridine Diphosphate Glucuronic Acid: A nucleoside diphosphate sugar which serves as a source of glucuronic acid for polysaccharide biosynthesis. It may also be epimerized to UDP iduronic acid, which donates iduronic acid to polysaccharides. In animals, UDP glucuronic acid is used for formation of many glucosiduronides with various aglycones. [NIH]

Urinary: Having to do with urine or the organs of the body that produce and get rid of urine. [NIH]

Urine: Fluid containing water and waste products. Urine is made by the kidneys, stored in the bladder, and leaves the body through the urethra. [NIH]

Urticaria: A vascular reaction of the skin characterized by erythema and wheal formation due to localized increase of vascular permeability. The causative mechanism may be allergy, infection, or stress. [NIH]

Vaccine: A substance or group of substances meant to cause the immune system to respond to a tumor or to microorganisms, such as bacteria or viruses. [NIH]

Vacuole: A fluid-filled cavity within the cytoplasm of a cell. [NIH]

Valerian: Valeriana officinale, an ancient, sedative herb of the large family Valerianaceae. The roots were formerly used to treat hysterias and other neurotic states and are presently used to treat sleep disorders. [NIH]

Vancomycin: Antibacterial obtained from Streptomyces orientalis. It is a glycopeptide related to ristocetin that inhibits bacterial cell wall assembly and is toxic to kidneys and the inner ear. [NIH]

Varicella: Chicken pox. [EU]

Vascular: Pertaining to blood vessels or indicative of a copious blood supply. [EU]

Vasculitis: Inflammation of a blood vessel. [NIH]

Vasoconstriction: Narrowing of the blood vessels without anatomic change, for which constriction, pathologic is used. [NIH]

Vasodilator: An agent that widens blood vessels. [NIH]

Vasomotor: 1. Affecting the calibre of a vessel, especially of a blood vessel. 2. Any element or agent that effects the calibre of a blood vessel. [EU]

Vein: Vessel-carrying blood from various parts of the body to the heart. [NIH]

Venlafaxine: An antidepressant drug that is being evaluated for the treatment of hot flashes in women who have breast cancer. [NIH]

Ventilation: 1. In respiratory physiology, the process of exchange of air between the lungs and the ambient air. Pulmonary ventilation (usually measured in litres per minute) refers to the total exchange, whereas alveolar ventilation refers to the effective ventilation of the alveoli, in which gas exchange with the blood takes place. 2. In psychiatry, verbalization of one's emotional problems. [EU]

Ventricle: One of the two pumping chambers of the heart. The right ventricle receives oxygen-poor blood from the right atrium and pumps it to the lungs through the pulmonary artery. The left ventricle receives oxygen-rich blood from the left atrium and pumps it to the body through the aorta. [NIH]

Ventricular: Pertaining to a ventricle. [EU]

Venules: The minute vessels that collect blood from the capillary plexuses and join together to form veins. [NIH]

Vertebrae: A bony unit of the segmented spinal column. [NIH]

Vertigo: An illusion of movement; a sensation as if the external world were revolving around the patient (objective vertigo) or as if he himself were revolving in space (subjective vertigo). The term is sometimes erroneously used to mean any form of dizziness. [EU]

Vestibular: Pertaining to or toward a vestibule. In dental anatomy, used to refer to the tooth surface directed toward the vestibule of the mouth. [EU]

Vestibule: A small, oval, bony chamber of the labyrinth. The vestibule contains the utricle and saccule, organs which are part of the balancing apparatus of the ear. [NIH]

Vestibulocochlear Nerve: The 8th cranial nerve. The vestibulocochlear nerve has a cochlear part (cochlear nerve) which is concerned with hearing and a vestibular part (vestibular nerve) which mediates the sense of balance and head position. The fibers of the cochlear nerve originate from neurons of the spiral ganglion and project to the cochlear nuclei (cochlear nucleus). The fibers of the vestibular nerve arise from neurons of Scarpa's ganglion and project to the vestibular nuclei. [NIH]

Vestibulocochlear Nerve Diseases: Diseases of the vestibular and/or cochlear (acoustic) nerves, which join to form the vestibulocochlear nerve. Vestibular neuritis, cochlear neuritis, and acoustic neuromas are relatively common conditions that affect these nerves. Clinical manifestations vary with which nerve is primarily affected, and include hearing loss, vertigo, and tinnitus. [NIH]

Veterinary Medicine: The medical science concerned with the prevention, diagnosis, and treatment of diseases in animals. [NIH]

Viral: Pertaining to, caused by, or of the nature of virus. [EU]

Virulence: The degree of pathogenicity within a group or species of microorganisms or viruses as indicated by case fatality rates and/or the ability of the organism to invade the tissues of the host. [NIH]

Virus: Submicroscopic organism that causes infectious disease. In cancer therapy, some viruses may be made into vaccines that help the body build an immune response to, and kill, tumor cells. [NIH]

Viscosity: A physical property of fluids that determines the internal resistance to shear forces. [EU]

Vitreous: Glasslike or hyaline; often used alone to designate the vitreous body of the eye (corpus vitreum). [EU]

Vitreous Body: The transparent, semigelatinous substance that fills the cavity behind the crystalline lens of the eye and in front of the retina. It is contained in a thin hyoid membrane and forms about four fifths of the optic globe. [NIH]

Vulgaris: An affection of the skin, especially of the face, the back and the chest, due to chronic inflammation of the sebaceous glands and the hair follicles. [NIH]

Wakefulness: A state in which there is an enhanced potential for sensitivity and an efficient responsiveness to external stimuli. [NIH]

White blood cell: A type of cell in the immune system that helps the body fight infection and disease. White blood cells include lymphocytes, granulocytes, macrophages, and others. [NIH]

Whooping Cough: A respiratory infection caused by Bordetella pertussis and characterized by paroxysmal coughing ending in a prolonged crowing intake of breath. [NIH]

Whooping Cough: A respiratory infection caused by Bordetella pertussis and characterized by paroxysmal coughing ending in a prolonged crowing intake of breath. [NIH]

Withdrawal: 1. A pathological retreat from interpersonal contact and social involvement, as may occur in schizophrenia, depression, or schizoid avoidant and schizotypal personality disorders. 2. (DSM III-R) A substance-specific organic brain syndrome that follows the cessation of use or reduction in intake of a psychoactive substance that had been regularly used to induce a state of intoxication. [EU]

X-ray: High-energy radiation used in low doses to diagnose diseases and in high doses to treat cancer. [NIH]

Zoster: A virus infection of the Gasserian ganglion and its nerve branches, characterized by discrete areas of vesiculation of the epithelium of the forehead, the nose, the eyelids, and the cornea together with subepithelial infiltration. [NIH]

INDEX

Procaine, 135, 144
Procyclidine, 67, 144
Progenitalis, 70, 144
Progressive, 123, 125, 139, 140, 144, 147
Promethazine, 4, 52, 76, 82, 83, 119, 145
Prone, 61, 145
Propolis, 70, 145
Propoxyphene, 31, 145
Propylene Glycol, 59, 145
Protective Agents, 117, 145
Protein S, 116, 145
Proteins, 64, 111, 113, 118, 121, 132, 138, 139, 141, 143, 145, 149
Protons, 132, 135, 145, 146
Proximal, 118, 144, 145
Proxy, 44, 145
Pruritus, 145
Psychiatric, 12, 14, 137, 145
Psychiatry, 3, 4, 17, 18, 20, 25, 29, 38, 44, 128, 145, 151, 155
Psychic, 137, 145, 149
Psychoactive, 145, 156
Psychomotor Performance, 11, 26, 30, 145
Psychophysiology, 52, 145
Psychosis, 23, 43, 113, 145
Public Policy, 91, 146
Publishing, 4, 7, 146
Pulmonary, 7, 116, 117, 146, 151, 155
Pulmonary Edema, 7, 146
Purpura, 32, 146
Pyrilamine, 59, 146
Q
Quaternary, 13, 15, 64, 146, 148
R
Radiation, 112, 129, 135, 136, 146, 154, 156
Radiation therapy, 146, 154
Radioactive, 131, 132, 146
Radiography, 119, 122, 146
Radioimmunotherapy, 146
Radiotherapy, 41, 146
Randomized, 3, 6, 10, 12, 15, 19, 24, 26, 36, 40, 126, 146
Ranitidine, 5, 62, 146
Ranitidine Hydrochloride, 5, 146
Reactivation, 144, 146
Reagent, 65, 127, 146
Reality Testing, 145, 147
Receptor, 13, 28, 59, 60, 62, 68, 109, 113, 120, 124, 125, 128, 131, 136, 139, 140, 147, 149, 152
Rectal, 41, 69, 147
Rectum, 113, 116, 124, 129, 134, 135, 147

Red Nucleus, 114, 147
Reductase, 137, 147
Refer, 1, 60, 121, 125, 128, 132, 136, 139, 145, 146, 147, 153, 155
Reflex, 128, 147
Reflux, 147, 151
Refractory, 17, 126, 147
Refractory cancer, 17, 147
Regimen, 27, 35, 126, 141, 147
Regurgitation, 51, 131, 147
Remission, 4, 136, 147
Renal failure, 123, 147
Research Design, 4, 147
Reserpine, 116, 147
Resorption, 129, 147
Respiratory distress syndrome, 27, 147
Respiratory Physiology, 147, 155
Retina, 68, 119, 140, 148, 156
Rheumatoid, 58, 70, 138, 143, 148
Rheumatoid arthritis, 58, 70, 138, 143, 148
Rhinitis, 59, 117, 119, 148, 154
Rigidity, 141, 143, 148
Ristocetin, 148, 154
Rod, 115, 148
S
Salicylate, 68, 124, 148
Saline, 15, 48, 148
Saliva, 33, 148
Salivary, 119, 124, 128, 148
Salivary glands, 119, 124, 128, 148
Salivation, 130, 148
Schizoid, 148, 156
Schizophrenia, 17, 148, 156
Schizotypal Personality Disorder, 148, 156
Scopolamine, 16, 67, 76, 115, 148
Screening, 44, 120, 148
Sebaceous, 123, 148, 156
Secobarbital, 8, 33, 40, 148
Secretion, 118, 119, 128, 132, 138, 140, 142, 146, 148
Sedative, 8, 10, 16, 31, 38, 59, 67, 69, 111, 115, 120, 136, 137, 145, 148, 154
Sedatives, Barbiturate, 148
Sediment, 149
Sedimentation, 69, 149
Seizures, 117, 120, 123, 141, 142, 149
Self Care, 109, 149
Semicircular canal, 134, 149
Sensitization, 36, 143, 149
Serologic, 133, 149
Serotonin, 111, 113, 129, 131, 139, 140, 147, 149

CPSIA information can be obtained at www.ICGtesting.com
Printed in the USA
LVOW021918270213

321893LV00001B/112/A